"The ICE Method profound   many
unconscious causes and soluti   in for
almost 20 years I can say easi   easeful
method I have used to date—   method
to anyone who suffers from   physical,
mental, or spiritual. I use ICE daily myself— a   for self-healing and wellness!"

 Kari Lyons-Price,
 President NCW Integrative Health Network

"For five decades I lived with constant fight/flight/freeze stress and anxiety, including frequent panic attacks. For the past two years, ICE has been an absolutely simple, safe and effective way to live calm and chip away at any of my personal baggage."

 Dennis Dyck, EFT Practitioner, Nanaimo, British Columbia

"Just after getting a college volleyball scholarship, I tore my ACL and meniscus. I used The ICE Method to calm my fears about my injury and my worries about the future of my volleyball career. I'm staying calm throughout the recovery and I feel it's helping my body to recover more quickly."

 Eliana Ali'ilima-Daley, Cascade High School

"I recommend some of my clients to work with Lars and they come back with very positive outcomes every time."

 Josette Pelletier, Co-founder, Inner Mountain Healing Art
 Craniosacral Therapy, Alexander Technique, Massage

"I found the ICE method to be an amazingly simple and incredibly effective process. I was sold immediately when I tried it on some neck pain that had not budged no matter what other methods and medications I had tried. Once I used ICE, the pain melted away and didn't return. I have also tried ICE on emotional issues with equal success."

 Tamara Staples. President, Fibromyalgia-ME/CFS Support Center.

"Lars Clausen understands the chemistry of calm. I've already used his simple ICE Method to bring calm to childhood issues that nothing else ever addressed so directly and effectively. Just after learning the ICE Method we had a serious illness in our family and I used The ICE Method to stay calm and present. I am a Mental Health Counselor, and I'll be integrating Memory Reconsolidation and The ICE Method into my work with war veterans and others with PTSD."

Janet Roberson, M Ed, LMHC

"I had to leave college because of crippling pain and illness. Three sessions of The ICE Method alleviated my stress and my pain. Thanks to The ICE Method, I'm back in school again, pain free!!!"

Naomi Ellingson, Western Washington University

"The ICE method has greatly facilitated me in my journey. It has helped calm down my nervous system and inflammation enough to allow my body to heal without looping through the same patterns of pain. I am more aware of the present moment, less anxious and have been enjoying the movement of my body. I overcame fibromyalgia. I am a success story!"

Roxanna Adams, Intuitive Empath, Winthrop WA

"We are fortunate for this book and the author's healing work, both grounded in the solid neuroscience of memory reconsolidation. In a very clear, simple and accessible manner, he connects breakthrough science with an effective healing practice - remarkably available to all. Of particular import is his critical distinction between the traditional counteractive therapy of building new habits, and the elegant simple process of changing peptides. This is a healing method that surely has a bright and strong future. Looking forward to more of this author's work. Highly recommended!"

John Neff, DMin, Life Coach, QiGong and Tai Chi Teacher

"Thank you for teaching me this incredibly simple approach to dealing with life's challenges. You've made our lives better."

Vicki Cash, RN

Memory Reconsolidation Applied

*Calm Your Past
to Live Your Future*

By Lars Clausen

www.ICEMethod.com
www.MemoryReconsolidation.org

Copyright © 2015 Lars C. Clausen
All Rights Reserved
ISBN: 978-1507831854

"I must be willing to give up what I am in order to become what I will be."
Albert Einstein

Contents

Foreword	ix
Introduction	xi
Part One	
1 – A Living Mom Memory	19
2 – Memory Reconsolidation	31
3 – Paying Attention	41
4 – The ICE Method	51
Part Two	
5 – Dad's Memory is Still Alive	61
6 – What Do You Really Want?	71
7 – ICE'ing the Download	87
8 – PTSD, Panic, Abuse, and Extreme Upsets	105
9 – Neuroplasticity and Neurogenesis	119
10 - Quantum	125
11 – A Spirit Side of Peptides	137
12 – Death	147
13 – Integrating ICE with Existing Methods	150
14 – Last Words	163
Workbook and Journal	167
Personal Sessions and Coaching	168
Author	169
Appendix – The Field	171
Disclaimer	179
Index	181
Endnotes	185

Foreword

Lars Clausen is the first person I have heard speak about Memory Reconsolidation; the concept of emotional memory being stored in peptides. When he first explained this concept to me, with my training as a medic as well as being a doctor of acupuncture and oriental medicine, what he spoke of made absolute sense to me.

I cannot think of a person I have ever encountered who has not had some "life-altering experience." Every experience in our lives has helped us become the people we now are.

Throughout time and cultures these events have been discussed in many ways. In classical Chinese medicine texts, the concept of memories being stored in the blood is discussed. In Native American traditions, it is believed that pieces of the soul can separate when one goes through a traumatic event. Some of these pieces can even get left behind when one "checks out" from an unbearable emotional event. In more recent times, there are discussions taking place of traumas being passed from one generation to the next not only in action, but also in cellular storage.

In my own life, I have experienced traumas. I have years of counseling and other experiences that have helped me learn to progress in a way that I am able to like the person that I am. Like many people though I still had certain triggers; events where I found myself questioning whether my response was related to what actually happened or was it just an automated response from training or conditioning. Half a year ago I did three sessions of The ICE Method with Lars. I was actually able to see what these automated responses were linked to and transform to a state of calm. In addition, the next time a similar event arose, I found that the feeling of calm was still present and that the triggered response of the past was no longer my first response.

Not only did Lars share this knowledge and gift with me, Lars now works with me at the Integrative Medical Clinic I am developing and where he is helping others through this work. When I feel it's appropriate, I offer clients sessions of acupuncture in combination with The ICE Method. Reconsolidating troubled memories at the same time I provide attention to the person's physical, emotional, and energetic needs has benefited many of my clients.

All of us have opportunities for challenging life lessons. Many of us have developed automatic responses that result in our belief that this is "just the way I work," or "just the way I respond to certain situations." Lars' work now provides an opportunity to change these automated responses, the ones we developed at a cellular level, in response to our life experiences.

Memory Reconsolidation Applied is a book that can help you create cellular change. It can help you facilitate your living with an emotional freedom in a more preferred state; a calmer state. You hold in your hands a book to reflect upon and apply the words and method to your own life experiences; a book that can help you change your life's patterned responses.

Dr. Catherine Freeman, DAOM
Doctor of Acupuncture and Oriental Medicine
Wellness Garden Integrative Medical Clinic
Chelan, Washington.

Introduction

In working with hundreds of people for a wide variety of emotional, physical and spiritual issues; people often asked me for a book on applying Memory Reconsolidation. You can find countless titles on the science of the brain and countless more on healing mind, body and spirit. Yet until now, no general book explained Memory Reconsolidation to the public and provided a simple method for using it in daily life. To date I know of only three books specifically about Memory Reconsolidation; a technical science compilation,[1] a psychotherapy application[2] and a book I published in 2013 to help people with fibromyalgia.[3]

I started this book many times and kept feeling blocked until I reached this single particular contribution I feel qualified to make.

**I can share the findings of Memory Reconsolidation
in a simple way, and I can offer an easy-to-learn process
for calming whatever upset emotions you have stored in your life.**

It does not matter how long ago the experiences happened or how far into the future your anxiety might reach. The intensity of your issue also does not matter. Memory Reconsolidation is the science of how experiences store as memories and how the stored emotion of even old memories can permanently change to calm.

**If there is no immediate truly physical threat
to your life in the present moment, you can turn off
your fight/flight/freeze response and reconsolidate
stored emotions to a permanent state of calm.**

You can use the simple ICE Method I share in this book, or you can integrate the findings of Memory Reconsolidation into your own already existing practices. What matters - what remains little known outside the laboratory - is the actual chemical process of how the emotions of memories store, activate and then reconsolidate. Know this process of Memory Reconsolidation, and you can free yourself from emotional reactivity to past experiences or future worries.

When I first read about the discovery of Memory Reconsolidation, I felt I had an explanation for the dramatic results I'd experienced using the Emotional Freedom Technique (EFT). I kept reading and learning, and ultimately I combined what I read about Memory Reconsolidation with the findings of neuroscientist Candace Pert.[4] Her decades of research showed how molecules called peptides store our emotions and inform the function of our mind and body.. She also showed that these peptide "information molecules" can form based on our emotional feelings. Aware of these two scientific discoveries and my prior experience with EFT, I created a method that follows the three steps of Memory Reconsolidation. I named this The ICE Method.

- The letter "**I**" stands for *Identify*. First you identify whatever memories, emotions and physical sensations relate to the issue. This activates the stored peptides that hold the upset.
- The letter "**C**" stands for *Calm*. If you can shift your emotional attention outside of the issue for a moment, then the memory can be reconsolidated. I've chosen to shift attention to a calm place because in the process we turn off our fight/flight/freeze system.
- The letter "**E**" stands for *Exchange* of the emotional peptide molecules. Crazy, but if you do the first two steps and then look back on what you originally identified, you will reconsolidate the original memory, the original emotion and the original sensations in the body. When you do this you replace the original peptide chemistry with calm chemistry – permanently. This is Memory Reconsolidation.

This is the very specific focus of this book
- To show the brain-level importance of Memory Reconsolidation for emotional, physical, and spiritual well-being.

Introduction

- To provide you a simple method for using Memory Reconsolidation in your daily life.

This book matters because Memory Reconsolidation opens a new door for healing emotional memory. Up until the discovery of Memory Reconsolidation in the year 2000, brain scientists believed our memories remained fixed and unchangeable. Until then therapists mostly offered ways to adapt and cope with the experiences of life. Memory Reconsolidation changed that belief in the laboratory. For a small but growing number, Memory Reconsolidation changes our view of mind and body. This book updates some commonly held beliefs about memory and emotion.

Given how many of us live with reactivity to stuck emotions and experiences, any available help would offer huge benefits.

How many of us in middle or elder age can still remember a parent's action from when we were kids and still recall an emotion of anger or fear or sadness? And how many of us can still feel these emotions in our bodies when we pay attention with our minds? Many of us, probably almost all of us, can. Even many healing practitioners find their lives contain stuck emotions that haven't dislodged after all levels of work and effort. Memory Reconsolidation offers an effective, speedy and durable answer to permanently replacing emotional upsets with calm.

In the year 2000, Karim Nader and Glenn Schafe[5] trained fear memories into four laboratory mice and then erased those fears. This was the discovery of Memory Reconsolidation that has given us a new understanding of how stored emotions can be replaced. Over 500 papers have so far been published about Memory Reconsolidation. Yet, with very few exceptions, the discovery remains only in the laboratory.

Since coming upon Nader's results in 2012, I have been captivated and transformed by Memory Reconsolidation. I have used The ICE Method with over 200 people dealing with a wide variety of issues from anxiety and panic to fibromyalgia and chronic pain. Most importantly, though, I have lived ICE since becoming aware of how Memory Reconsolidation happens in our brain.

After more than two years of experience with this technique, I now welcome the arrival of an upset emotion. After a lifetime of reacting to upsets, I now see them as opportunities. When they show up, I first check to see if I face an immediate physical threat. If not, I use ICE.

When I first became aware of ICE, I used it almost constantly. Once I experienced this ability to get calm and to ICE stored upsets, I discovered how much of my life had held upsets. I used to feel upset if things didn't go my way. I used to feel upset if other people arrived late. I used to worry what people thought of me or my actions. I could remember childhood patterns that still carried a charge. I started ICE'ing *everything*. Within a month of starting to experiment with this new ICE Method, my baseline began transforming from an underlying anger to a grounding in calm. I went from being a mostly reactive person with periods of calm, to a mostly calm person with interruptions to that calm state.

I find it difficult to express the enormous and fundamental change I have experienced with this transformation to calm. Even though I had been a pastor years earlier and even though I had been interested in healing for a number of years I had no idea, no sense, of how completely I had lived in reaction to stored emotional upsets. Only when I started reconsolidating my upsets and began transforming my baseline to calm, did I realize how much these stored emotions and reactivity had dominated my actions and my being.

Bringing calm to my emotional past has transformed my life from "mostly reactivity" to "mostly inner peace." I have a much better sense now of what the spiritual traditions mean by "non-attachment." As reactivity has given way to calm, the horizons of peace, love and compassion have grown wider in my life. I've wanted these qualities all my life, but the path has been mysterious. Discovering that The ICE Method provides a direct process for expanding our spiritual awareness came as an unexpected benefit. Emotional upsets still occur in my life, but much less frequently than before. And when they do, I use The ICE Method to reconsolidate the upset into calm.

Sharing the Memory Reconsolidation process so others can enjoy greater well-being has been a huge joy for me these past few years. I feel thrilled to share my experience now in this book. So whether you offer healing to others or you seek healing for yourself, whether you live as a spiritual leader or a spiritual seeker, a scientist or a poet, I wish for you your own discovery of Memory Reconsolidation and its usefulness for your life.

Workbook, Website, and Personal Sessions

If you find yourself connecting to this ICE Method and to the experience of calm, you may want more. At my website, you'll find many resources, including the workbook I published to go along with this book.

Website: **www.MemoryReconsolidationApplied.com**
Workbook: **Memory Reconsolidation Applied:** *The ICE Method Workbook and Journal*

I offer in-person and online ICE Method sessions and training at the Wellness Garden Integrative Medical Clinic in Chelan, Washington. For more information visit TheICEMethod.com.

Notes before beginning

I am not a doctor or certified healthcare provider. I am an engineer, pastor, author, unicyclist, Guinness World Record Holder who cares about body, mind, and spirit. Read the disclaimer in the appendix of the book. You are responsible for whatever you take from this book and however you use it.

Privacy matters to me. The stories in this book remain true to the actual experiences, but names and circumstances have been changed in this book to maintain confidentiality.

Part One

Learning The ICE Method

1 – A Living Mom Memory

"I feel the anger in my stomach." Shock and disbelief spread across Ben's face.

"But I've already done so much therapy to deal with my mother. Years I worked on this. How can I still feel this anger?"

Ben and I have been friends since my days of unicycling across the United States. I have not seen him in many years. Tonight my wife Anne and I have stopped to stay at his home, en route to a conference.

After dinner Ben had asked me, "What's this ICE Method stuff you do now?"

Whenever I have time I prefer to show people The ICE Method rather than explain it. Ben and I have the whole evening for visiting and catching up so I had replied by asking Ben to choose a parent and let me know if he felt an emotion when he thought of either of them.

"Anger," Ben had said, "I used to feel so much anger toward my mom. But I've done a lot of years of counseling, and I'm over the anger now."

"Good," I had responded, "But do me a favor and pay attention to that anger for a moment. And when you pay attention, notice if you feel any sensation in your body as you pay attention to the anger."

That was the moment Ben's face turned to disbelief.

"How can I still feel anger in my stomach?" Ben asks me again.

"Because you never removed the actual stored chemistry of your anger," I tell Ben. "Your therapy probably gave you some excellent understanding about you and your mom. And you probably learned ways to deal with your anger rather than reacting like you did before therapy."

"Yes, that's exactly what it did for me."

"And that's a fantastic benefit for your life. Emotions store as chemistry in our brain, though, and most therapy never touches that old chemistry. That's why you can still feel the anger in your stomach when you pay attention to it in your mind."

I continue, "Changing this stored chemistry was the discovery of Memory Reconsolidation. In the year 2000, researchers discovered when you access a memory you get about a four-hour window to transform the stored chemical emotion of that memory. If you know what to do during that window of time, you can transform upset memories to the emotion of calm. That's what I help people do."

"Really? You can just go into a person's brain and change out upset emotions?"

"Pretty much. Actually I lead people through The ICE Method, and they change out their own emotions. They become non-attached to the emotions they've been reacting to, even all the way back to childhood. For most people, it's different from anything they've experienced before.

"I can show you how it works." I offer. "Maybe you can get your mother out of your stomach."

"Okay, let's give it a try," Ben agrees.

"If you think about your mom," I begin, "what do you feel was her primary emotion when she wasn't calm? Was it anger, fear, sadness, or something else?"

My friend reflects for a moment. "She always acted so angry around us kids, but underneath I feel like she had a lot of fear."

"Okay, so as you observe this about your mom, notice what emotion you feel in reaction to your mom's emotion."

Immediately now, "Anger. So much anger."

"And you feel this in your stomach?"

"Yes."

"Do you feel it anywhere else in your body?"

"My shoulders and my neck," he notes with another look of surprise. "I have a lot of ongoing neck problems."

"What we're doing right now is the first step of The ICE Method. We're *identifying* some of the stored emotions you have about your mom. You became aware of your emotion of anger, and also two locations in your body that you notice when you pay attention to your anger.

"Okay, so now see if any specific memories or experiences rise to the surface as you pay attention to your mother, to the anger, and to your stomach, shoulders, and neck. Imagine maybe that you're walking through the display at a garage sale, just seeing what's there. We're not digging holes in the lawn to discover any deep meanings; we're just walking through the yard and allowing memories to activate. We're checking for the emotions, the sensations in your body and specific memories."

I wait a moment. "Got some?"

"I'm remembering stuff from when I was a kid."

"Okay, good. You just completed the "I," the identify of The ICE Method. You identified the upset emotion of anger. Then you identified the location in your body; that you feel it in your stomach, neck and shoulders. And the third part you identified are these memories that showed up when you paid attention to the anger emotion. According to Memory Reconsolidation, these emotions will stay activated for the next four hours. If you don't reconsolidate them they will "reglue" in the same old way. Up to now, whenever you've felt this anger emotion, you've never done a conscious process to replace the anger with another emotion. The therapy you did never caused the chemical reconsolidation of these old anger emotions. If you want, we can do this right now."

"Sure. But I thought that happened already in therapy – that's why I spent all those years working on this."

"Therapy gave you great tools to deal with your anger. But therapy didn't remove the stored chemistry of that anger. If you want, we can remove that anger chemistry right now, and replace it with calm."

"Let's do it."

"Now the next part of The ICE Method is the "C;" getting you to the *calm* state. This is all chemistry. Emotions store in the synapses that connect brain cells. The emotions store as peptide molecules. Peptides are short proteins; people call these 'information molecules.' You just activated the old peptides, and now you'll get to a calm state and create some calm peptide molecules."

"The brain scientists really know the brain works this way?"

"Over 500 research papers have been published about Memory Reconsolidation.[6] It's mostly still just a laboratory discovery, but once I understood Memory Reconsolidation, it became much easier to help people with their upsets, their pain and even sometimes, their spiritual journeys.

"There's another scientist named Candace Pert.[7] On her own she published over 250 papers. She studied peptides molecules, what she called the "molecules of emotion." When you have an emotion, a peptide forms. Your emotion turns into a chemical signal that affects both your mind and your body."

I continue. "So, let's see what happens. If you'll just look at the corner of that picture frame on your wall over there, you'll shift your conscious attention from your anger about your mom to that one single point. It turns out whatever you pay attention to, you create a chemical signal and your body responds to support you. If you focus on the anger toward your mom, your stomach hurts. If you focus on a single point, there's not much for your body or your mind to do. You literally start to relax."

After a moment I invite my friend to shift his focus to the corner of the frame of another picture on his wall. After he observes this for a moment I help him go deeper into this calm feeling.

"Okay, so now notice that between the two points you observed, you can imagine an empty space. There's a wall behind this space, of course, but between any two points you choose, you can always imagine the empty space between them. Just observe this empty space."

I let Ben observe this empty space for a moment and then explain. "When we observe something in our outside world, our body and mind react to whatever we pay attention to. If we observe something we perceive as stressful or dangerous, then our body responds with fight/flight/freeze stress. That's what happens when you observe a memory of your mom – even though the memory is from your childhood, your fight/flight/freeze activates right now. You feel that in your stomach.

"But if we consciously observe nothing, then with our mind we confirm that nothing in our outside world needs a response from us in this immediate moment. When our body receives this *'do not respond'* message, then our fight/flight/freeze stress response turns off. Our body relaxes into a state of rest and restoration. Do you feel the difference?"

"Yes, I do," he says to me. "My whole body just relaxed. And my shoulders just dropped a couple of inches."

"Everyone I work with loves this feeling. Just enjoy it. This calm space feels different for different people. Some people feel their skin tingle, others feel their head decompress or their jaw relax. For me I get a lowering feeling in my chest whenever I'm aware of this calm space.

"Over a thousand chemical reactions take place in your body when you switch from fight/flight/freeze to calm. In this calm place, all the cells of your body focus on healing, rest, and restoration. Literally your cells become better able to take in energy and get rid of waste. Cells can communicate better between each other. Even your DNA strands can begin to repair if they've been under a lot of stress.[8]

"This calm makes a great place to live your life from. It's part of why meditation, yoga, massage, and all sorts of relaxation techniques help so much. You can use other ways besides this two-point and calm space method. I like it because it's so simple. Almost everyone experiences calm when they do this little process."[9]

"I really like this." Ben looks noticeably calmer than just moments before when he had his mind on his mother and the pain in his stomach.

"We could just stop here," I tell him, "but if we do the "E" part of ICE, the *exchange*, that's when we can actually replace some of your old stored anger peptides.

"This exchange of peptides is the actual Memory Reconsolidation of your activated brain synapses. Just observe back on what you activated about your mom, the memories that came up, the emotion of anger, and the feeling in your stomach, back, and neck."

I watch Ben focusing as he pays attention to his memories. "It may seem crazy, but Memory Reconsolidation is this simple. The activated synapses have this four-hour window where you can replace the old emotional peptides you stored for all these decades. So look back on exactly what you identified. Let me know what feels the same and what feels different."

Ben sits in his chair and observes what he feels now, paying attention to an important part of his life.

"Well, my stomach feels calm now. But I can still feel tightness in my shoulders and neck. The big memory that first showed up feels weird now. I don't have any anger when I think of it. It just feels like something that happened, but I don't feel any emotion about it." He pauses. "Now some different memories are showing up. These don't feel calm."

"So you reconsolidated at least some of your old stored emotional chemistry. You replaced it with these peptides that carry the message of calm. When your first memory turned calm, then your attention became aware of other memories."

"I can't believe that first experience feels calm now. That's been a big one since I was a little kid."

"This happens for almost everyone when they use The ICE Method. And this is all you need to know to start using ICE. Knowing the discovery of Memory Reconsolidation gives you a really powerful tool. You know what you're looking for, and you know when you've gotten a result. Then you just take whatever shows up next and use ICE again. We've got something like 80 billion brain cells connected by trillions of synapse connections. So you'll find more things to ICE! Use it whenever something shows up that doesn't feel calm.

"After a couple years of using The ICE Method for myself, I still find things showing up sometimes that don't feel calm. But I've done Memory Reconsolidation so much that I totally trust it. It's very dependable and very repeatable. So I just ICE whatever shows up in my life now, and then I have a new part of my life that's calm."

Ben serves as a pastor in a small congregation, just like I used to many years ago. "I work with so many people where their basic issues are emotional. This seems like it could be such a useful tool for them."

"Plus," I add, "it lasts."

"How do you know it lasts?"

"Because once the memory reconsolidates it's just like any other memory. The emotion of memories stay that way unless they get reconsolidated."

"Think of it this way," I continue; "Your old emotions have been stuck there for decades. They'd be stuck there for a lifetime unless you use some intentional process like ICE and transform them to calm. So, now that you've reconsolidated this memory to a calm emotion, you'd have to do another intentional process if you wanted to switch out the calm emotion that you just created. If your old emotions can stay stuck forever, these new ones will too. There's a laboratory experiment they did with people testing a fear reaction. After they reconsolidated their fears, they tested them again a year later, and the fear response had not returned. From everything I've experienced, Memory Reconsolidation can bring permanent calm to old upset memories."[10]

I ask Ben, "Are you up for doing another round or two of ICE? You said some other memories showed up now, and you still feel tension in your neck and shoulders. We can stop anytime you want, but I always like to continue until people feel as calm as possible."

Ben agrees, and we start another round. Three more times he has new memories show up. Each round goes a bit quicker than before as he becomes aware of the calm space more quickly and naturally. After the last round, he tells me everything feels calm.

"If you observe your mother now, and the emotion of anger you started with, what shows up for you now?"

Ben sits for a moment. "Well, this is strange. I actually feel compassion for her. I feel like she did the best she was able to do. I don't feel any more anger."

"Not bad for an hour." I smile. "Tomorrow you might feel something else show up about your mother that's not calm. If something shows up, it will be different from whatever memories you activated tonight. Memory Reconsolidation works on exactly the synapses you activate. If something new shows up, it doesn't mean tonight's reconsolidation didn't work. It means you became aware of something new or different, something that didn't surface tonight. You have 80 billion brain cells and a lifetime of memories. I'd be surprised if you didn't come across other upsets in your life. Whatever arises from now on – if you wish – you can use The ICE Method and bring it to calm.

"This is amazing stuff," Ben says quietly.

"The only exception is a true immediate physical threat. In that case you'd be running or fighting and not thinking about calm. That's what your fight/flight/freeze stress response is made to respond to. Immediate physical danger is actually the only thing it's made for. Most of us just get mixed up and go into fight/flight/freeze for things that aren't physical dangers, including past memories and future worries. If you use ICE, you can be calm anytime except during an immediate physical danger."

"Wow," Ben says. He's thinking again. "You said it's been slow getting people introduced to this ICE Method. I can't believe people aren't lined up at your house."

"Me too," I laugh. "I had my own upset emotions about that for a while. I felt anger that people weren't trying ICE. And then I felt sad that I wasn't making a big splash with ICE. I kept paying attention to the anger and sadness until I ICE'd them to calm. And then I had to ICE my fear that maybe I'd never find a way to share this and make a living from it. Along the way, I've felt this tremendous sadness as I become more and more aware of the trauma so many of us live with. When that sadness arises, I let myself feel it and then ICE myself back to calm. After all that ICE'ing, I'm pretty much calm about where I'm at right now. I'm a lot closer to feeling non-attached to results. When new emotions catch me, I ICE them as I become aware of them. Who knows, maybe a big part of developing ICE is just for me to become more calm about my own life."

"That makes sense, but I still wonder why it hasn't taken off?"

"It could be I'm just a moron about business and communication." I laugh again. "But maybe ICE is taking a long time to catch on because it's so different from how we normally try to change our life."

"Yeah, it's crazy to believe this just happened. But it does make sense the way you described what happened in my brain and how this stuff can change."

"It does make sense, but I also think a lot of us feel so strongly reactive, we can't imagine life without our upsets. In fact, if you think about it, that anger emotion you had as a kid probably helped you survive your childhood."

"That's true for sure. I've actually felt grateful that I stayed angry and stuck up for myself as a kid. I didn't get swallowed up by all the craziness in my house. My brother and my sister weren't so lucky."

"Then at some point maybe you realized that you didn't need to be the angry boy to survive anymore. Maybe you realized what it was costing you to keep being the angry one. That might have been why you went to see your counselor."

"I hadn't made that exact connection, but yes, my life wasn't working very well when I started counseling. And my counselor and I did address my mom stuff during a lot of those sessions."

"So tonight, when you reconsolidated your stored anger emotions about your mom, you actually let go of your strongest survival tool from your childhood, your anger power toward your mom. And you must have felt ready to do that tonight or you wouldn't have wanted to try ICE. You were open to living from a more calm place. I think maybe a lot of people believe their emotional upsets are their survival tools."

I share a story with Ben, "Not long ago I was doing ICE with a woman after her house burned down. Her husband was there, but he didn't want to try ICE. He told me he needed his anger to deal with the insurance agents and all the stuff he had to go through after the fire. I told him that was fine and started to show his wife how to identify, calm and exchange her experience about the fire. After a little bit, the husband interrupted and asked what had just happened to him. Turns out he'd been following along with his wife's process and reconsolidated a part of his own anger."

Ben asks, "Did he get angry with you for taking away his anger?"

"He was pretty stunned for a while, but then he got real interested. At the end I asked if I could make a video of his experience to share with others. He told me no way. He didn't do public speaking.

"By that time we'd been visiting and ICE'ing for over an hour, and he was feeling calm about every aspect of his home burning to ashes. But the thought of making a video sparked a big charge. He could tell me the exact class in college and exactly what happened that was still such an upset memory. We ICE'd that to calm in about three minutes. Then I asked him to imagine what it would feel like to make that video and he said, 'Feels fine. I'm completely calm. Let's do it right now.' So we did. He stayed calm even when we started the video and he began talking."

"Maybe you need to be a public-speaking coach," Ben jokes. "Or maybe you just need to find the people who are ready to have calm in their lives. You don't have a counseling credential do you?"

"No. A Masters in engineering. A Masters in divinity. Nothing in medicine, or counseling or social work."

"I know you don't want to be a pastor again, but what about becoming a counselor?"

"There might be a way forward like that. Maybe a counseling degree would be helpful. I want to help people know that science now understands how upset emotions can transform permanently to calm. And I want to show people that this ICE Method is a simple way of reconsolidating your life to calm."

"So no one else is already doing this?"

"Now that I understand Memory Reconsolidation, I can look at other healing techniques and see how Memory Reconsolidation is happening when people are healing from their emotional traumas. I think lots of new developments are ahead, but so far I only know of two other places that are developing methods based specifically on the discovery of Memory Reconsolidation. One is a group of psychotherapists, and they call it Coherence Therapy.[11] The other fellow has become a friend of mine. He's developing what he's calling NeuroMastery Academy.[12] He's also having great success with the people who learn his techniques. We Skype every week or so and share ideas. Nice to have a friend as excited as me about applying Memory Reconsolidation."

Ben listens carefully. "Maybe what you need is a study."

"I actually do already have some results. I told you my first book on Memory Reconsolidation was *Fibromyalgia Relief*. I decided to write it because I did a study with 33 fibromyalgia patients. Eighty percent of them had zero pain after a single session.[13]"

"What's happening with the book?"

"A few people are reading it, and some people are having sessions with me. Those that use it are getting results. Apparently it's not an obvious choice to associate fibromyalgia with emotions and consciousness.

"Once a person tries ICE, then they have a choice: whether or not they want to make Memory Reconsolidation a tool for their whole life. Those who adopt ICE start shifting from reactivity toward freedom. I keep looking for a way to have more people know about Memory Reconsolidation. But the truth is, every time I watch this transformation happen, I feel like I'm on top of the world. I love standing alongside a person when their life opens up in this new and freer way."

"You're still a pastor Lars."

"Yeah, I think there's still some of the old pastor in me. I feel that way now, with what you experienced tonight about your mom. If I never get any further than helping one person at a time – I'll be okay with that. At the same time, though, I know this could make a difference for so many more people."

Ever since I've known Ben he's been a practically oriented person. When we first met, he had helped me arrange speaking locations during my unicycle tour. Now he keeps pushing me, trying to find a way forward for me.

"So, I don't have fibromyalgia." Ben says, "Do you mostly help people with fibromyalgia?"

"I chose writing about fibromyalgia because it's one of the diseases where even the medical establishment sees a frequent emotional connection to the symptoms. It seemed like an easy place to start sharing The ICE Method. But I work with all sorts of people, everything from fear of spiders to chronic back pain, panic attacks, neuropathy, upset stomachs. Mom and Dad emotions like yours show up often."

"Maybe it's just going to take more time," Ben says.

"And maybe," I say "it needs to be the right time for me, just like for the people I work with. The Buddhists and a lot of other traditions emphasize non-attachment. Christians don't talk about it much, but more than once Jesus advised giving away our riches. The more I use The ICE Method, the more I am beginning to see it as a scientific method of become non-attached: A really simple, dependable, mechanical way.

I say to Ben, "I know it's a big deal that you came to this calm place about your mom. I didn't know that you'd get here tonight, but I'm not surprised either. And now you are 'non-attached' to these specific emotions you used to hold about your mother. That gives you some new freedom in your life. What happened is not a mystery. You know what you did and you know how you became non-attached. You know chemistry changed in your brain, and you know that science now understands that process. You can use this for the rest of your life if you choose."

There have been many sessions I didn't want to end, enjoying watching a person as they reconsolidate and transform. We've been sitting a long time. Anne and Ben's wife return from a walk in town. Our conversation shifts.

After breakfast the next morning, Anne and I get ready to depart. When we walk out to the car I open my box of *Fibromyalgia Relief* copies and give one to Ben.

"I'm working on a more general book about using The ICE Method, but the science of Memory Reconsolidation is in here, and how to do ICE. After our visit last night, I think you'll enjoy it." I thank Ben for his ideas about sharing The ICE Method, and he thanks me for showing him how to bring calm to his past.

As we drive away I wonder what Ben will do with The ICE Method. Will it become core to his life as it has for me? Or will it prove too different, too strange, too unbelievable - that the brain and body can transform so easily and with such a simple process?

2 – Memory Reconsolidation

"Can you help my husband with spiders?"

We start our third Skype session together, working on Mary's fibromyalgia. She lives in Texas, halfway across the country. The pain in her legs, her most painful symptom, feels markedly better than when we started.

"I'd like him to see how EFT works."

"Sure. "I am still half a year from finding out about Memory Reconsolidation. I've taken advanced training in EFT (Emotional Freedom Technique),[14] and the results working with people have taken me by surprise. As an engineer, I don't understand the mechanism behind the healing, but I can't deny the results people experience. Mary had been feeling constantly exhausted with significant pain in her joints. She has a lot more energy now, and her physical pain has lessened. She stands up and moves aside to let James take a seat in front of their computer screen.

"Tell me about the spiders," I invite.

"Spiders have terrified me since I was a kid. We had a basement shed. It was really dark in there and filled with cobwebs. My dad made me clean that basement every spring when I was little. I still see that basement clearly in my mind."

In EFT, you usually have the person rate their intensity. I don't even bother with James. His childhood upset is still clearly a ten out of ten, even though James must be in his sixties now. EFT then has you tap on a series of acupressure points on your head and upper body. While you do this, you repeat what you're upset about and also say, "Even though I have this fear of spiders, I deeply and completely accept myself."

EFT has various explanations for why it works – energy meridians, piezoelectric effects, body polarity and more. Back when I was doing EFT I was constantly trying to understand how it worked. While the explanations all interested me, I still found the theories more mysterious than mechanical. Yet, mystery or no, fifteen minutes later James was visualizing a spider on his computer keyboard and reporting, "I'm feeling calm. No problem."

"Okay, now I want you to make a video in your mind from when you were a child. Start from when your father ordered you to clean the basement, through opening the door and until you're finished with the job. Stop at the first moment you feel something not calm."

James closes his eyes and starts his mental movie. "When I get to the door of the basement and have to open it, I don't feel calm."

"Okay, exactly what do you notice in your mind that doesn't feel calm?"

"There were spiders crawling all over the inside of that door. I hated that door."

We tap through another round of EFT. "Even though I'm remembering all the spiders on the basement door, even though I'm feeling this old fear, I deeply and completely accept myself."

The next time James runs his spider movie, he gets all the way through feeling completely calm.

"Excellent, now you see how it works. This is what your wife is doing for her fibromyalgia. We do EFT on whatever doesn't feel calm when she pays attention to her emotions and memories about living with fibromyalgia. Sometimes taking a single big memory from charged to calm can change the whole way that the body experiences pain."

"That seems so strange. Mary's been in pain for so many years." James tells me. "But it also feels unbelievable to be feeling calm about spiders right now."

Three years later I am checking in with Mary, seeing how she's feeling.

"James wants to talk with you," Mary tells me after we visit a bit.

"Hi Lars. I wanted to tell you about our vacation. We were visiting my son, and he had this corner of his yard that was all messy. Everything else was picked up except there. He told me he couldn't do it because he'd seen spiders in that pile of leaves and sticks. I told him I'd clean it up for him.

"He was shocked – he's known about my fear of spiders all his life. He couldn't believe I don't feel afraid anymore."

"That's great." Three years later, and the results still hold for James.

"I think I passed my spider fear onto my son. I told him a couple different times he should call you."

"Sure, he can call me anytime. I haven't heard from him yet."

"Well, I'm pretty sure he thinks it's impossible for him to get rid of his spider fear."

"Yeah, I think most of us believe our emotions will stay stuck forever. You amazed me when you had such interest in trying EFT out three years ago."

"I'm glad I did. A few weeks ago I found a dead spider in the living room. Before you helped me, I would have gotten the vacuum cleaner to get rid of it. I would have stayed as far away as possible, even though it was already dead. This time I just got a scrap of paper, scooped it up and dropped it out the back door. I never would have done that before. Who would have known it could be so easy to not be afraid of spiders. I'll keep telling my son about you."

Before I develop The ICE Method, I will make use of EFT for three years, first personally and then more and more with others. The more it works, the more I wonder how it works.

A half year after helping a woman get over her fear of snakes, she shows up at my door, shaking a glass jar in her hand. She lives on an orchard, and the many rattlesnakes on the property had terrified her. Inside the jar the tails of five or six snakes rattle. She's excited to show me and also completely calm.

"Look," she says with glee. "I'm not scared of snakes anymore!"

Results like this happen all the time with EFT.

Then three years ago I come upon this mention of Memory Reconsolidation in a book about neuroscience. The Synaptic Self was written in 2002 by Joseph LeDoux:

> Studies of fear conditioning have also revived interest in a strange but possibly very significant phenomenon in memory research – reconsolidation. The recent discovery by Karim Nader and Glenn Schafe in my lab, is that protein synthesis…seems necessary for a recently activated memory to be kept as a memory. That is, if you

take a memory out of storage you have to make new proteins (you have to restore, or reconsolidate it) in order for it to remain a memory.[15]

"If you take a memory out of storage, you have to make new proteins in order for it to remain a memory." I have been searching for exactly this, the key to the puzzle of why EFT provides emotional and physical results. In all the time to come I never find it said more clearly anywhere else.

This paragraph from Joseph LeDoux describes what occurs in the brain when the upsets transform to calm – Memory Reconsolidation. When I read this paragraph, I know I've found the key that explains what I observe when using EFT. It will take a bit more time to unpack this key. When I do it will lead me to creating a new healing method.

This book shares how to change upset emotions to calm. Although the discovery was made in the year 2000, very few people outside the laboratory have yet become aware of Memory Reconsolidation. If you take some time in this section of the book, you'll get a feel for the science of what's happening in your brain. I've had many people ask me in all seriousness; "Is this all there is to it?"

Yes. This is the process that science says happens in our brain when stored upsets become permanently calm. You'll find the process simple, but you'll probably also find it counterintuitive. We did not grow up thinking this way. Play with the information here until it becomes familiar to you. Play with The ICE Method until it becomes comfortable. If you do, you will transform your life.

The primary problem preventing the calming of upsets.

Most people on this planet seem to believe past emotions remain permanently stored for as long as we live. If we believe the emotion of a stored memory can change, we mostly believe it's going to be a hard, unpredictable and often mysterious process.

The key of Memory Reconsolidation

"If you take a memory out of storage, you have to make new proteins in order for it to remain a memory."

It helps to know a few basics of how neuroscientists picture the brain storing emotions. Put as simply as I know how – when you have an experience, you store the *content* of that experience and you also store the *emotion* you feel at the time of the experience.[16]

It's helpful to envision the content of a memory being stored in a collection of brain cells that hold the memory.[17] The emotion of the memory stores at the junctions of the wiring that connect brain cells. These junction points are called *synapses*.

- **When you feel an emotion you create a peptide molecule.** This peptide is made from amino acids, just like any other protein. This peptide matches your emotion. It also provides the instruction for how your body should react – with happiness perhaps, or maybe anger, fear, or sadness. (Definition: A peptide is the same as a protein, just a short one instead of a long one.)
- **These emotion peptides also stores at the synapses in your brain.** As the original event becomes a memory, these peptides store at the connections between brain cells, at the synapses.
- **Later, when we recall a memory, we reactivate this original emotional peptide molecule.**
- **When the original emotional molecule reactivates, it influences our body again in the present moment**. The influence in the present moment will feel similar to whatever emotion you stored when the memory first happened long ago. If we felt fear many years ago when the experience happened, we'll trigger our fight/flight/freeze stress response and feel fear again when we recall the old memory.

A brief note: One of the most important books I've read has the great title *Molecules of Emotion*.[18] Candace Pert's work opened a whole new world of understanding for me, including how our emotions create peptides. These peptides then coordinate and control our brain, our body and even our immune system. Candace Pert lived her life with both a personal and scientific passion for probing the mind/body connection. If you're not yet aware of Pert's work, you'll probably find it a life-changer. I became aware of *Molecules of Emotion* only a few months before first reading about Memory Reconsolidation. Pert's work on peptides, combined with my experiences of using EFT tapping, helped me latch onto Memory Reconsolidation. Combining these influences I felt I had found a powerful key to improving our emotional, physical, and spiritual well-being. A couple quotes from Candace Pert:

> Emotional states or moods are produced by the various [peptides], and what we experience as an emotion or a feeling is also a mechanism for activating a particular neuronal circuit – simultaneously throughout the brain and body – which generates a behavior involving the whole creature, with all the necessary physiological changes that behavior would require.[19]
>
> We can no longer think of the emotions as having less validity than physical material substance, but instead must see them as cellular signals that are involved in the process of translating information into physical reality.[20]

Pert doesn't make these assertions just because she likes the sound of them. She published over 250 scientific papers in her lifetime, all about peptides. And based on a lifetime of detailed experiments and passionate inquiry, she sees that our emotions are translating information into physical reality.

If you find a way to deal with stored emotions, you change physical reality.

This is why the finding of Memory Reconsolidation made such a profound impact on me – if you change your stored emotions, you change almost everything about your life. Let's get back to developing this understanding of Memory Reconsolidation. Let's look at memory.

Say a memory takes a thousand brain cells to store the content of the memory, or maybe it's a million brain cells. Whatever the number, these brain cells are connected via wiring between the brain cells. Where the wires connect to each other is called a synapse. And where does the glue come from to wire the memory? From the peptides that formed in response to your emotions.

Memory Reconsolidation discovered that every time you recall a memory into your conscious awareness, you have to reglue that memory for it to remain a memory.

Why do stuck emotions stay so stuck?

Emotions appear stuck because we keep recalling the same emotion every time we recall the old memory. Unless we know of a process to transform that stored emotion, it will not ever change.

Recall a very happy childhood birthday party, and you will likely also recall and feel again that emotion of happiness. Recall a childhood abuse, and you will likely feel again the fear or the anger you originally felt at the time of the long-ago abuse.

If we don't know how Memory Reconsolidation works, then we will have no idea we need to access a different emotional peptide to replace our old stored upset emotion. Ben didn't know this so he kept feeling the anger emotions toward his mother for all the decades since his childhood. James didn't know this so he kept feeling his fear of spiders that he developed while a little kid.

There exists a window of time during which activated memories get reglued. Most researchers seem to think this window of time stays open for about four hours. Researchers are still investigating whether all activated memories reconsolidate, or whether reconsolidation only takes place when an emotion is transformed.[21] Based on my experience with hundreds of people, I think every memory that gets activated needs to reconsolidate or restabilize.

The big difference is whether you restabilize a memory with the same old emotions from the original memory, or whether you reconsolidate the memory with different emotional peptides – and transform the memory.

Emotions appear stuck for a lifetime because we mostly keep restabilizing memories in the same exact way, over and over again for our entire lifetime.

What normally happens is this: Since you feel the emotion of the original memory when you recall it, you will normally react to that emotion throughout your body as well as your mind. This old molecule will be all that's available to reglue the old memory. And that's what happens, the old memory reglues with the same old emotion. Result: Ben and James and most of us on the planet continue to feel the same emotions about our old memories. Unless we find a way to intervene we usually keep regluing our activated memories with the same original glue, the same emotion as when we first experienced the event. Memory Reconsolidation offers us a tool to change how the emotional content of a memory gets restabilized.

See how this works by using the example of an automobile accident, or any other emotional memory. The *content* of an automobile accident includes things like the color of the car that hits you, the time it takes for the emergency vehicles to show up, your particular injuries, etc. The *emotion* of the automobile accident is the fear or the anger or sadness or other emotion you feel. And when you recall an automobile accident, even years later, you usually feel the original emotion you first felt at the time of the experience. This emotion triggers your fight/flight/freeze stress response even though no actual danger exists from the past memory.

Before I became aware of Memory Reconsolidation, while I was still using EFT tapping; I helped a woman suffering from severe fibromyalgia pain.

Sarah tells me she has hurt with fibromyalgia for many years. "They only diagnosed me five years ago," she says, "but I've been having these pains for forty years."

"Do you remember when this pain began? Do you remember anything especially significant happening around that time?"

"Sure. I was in my early twenties. I know right when the pain started. I was in a car accident in Nebraska." Sarah stops and when she starts again her voice trembles. "A good friend of mine was killed. I recovered but I had a shoulder pain that never went away. Since that time the pains have been adding up and getting worse over the years. Now my legs feel painful all the time. A lot of times I can't even walk up the stairs in my house. I have to crawl."

"When you pay attention to the memory of the car accident now, do your pain symptoms stay the same or do they feel different?"

Sarah gets a look of surprise on her face. "They just started feeling much worse. My neck just got really sore and tight"

I still feel surprised myself, but this mind-body connection between stored emotions and physical sensations in our body keeps showing up again and again.

Over five succeeding sessions Sarah uses the tapping method of EFT. During the second session she becomes calm about the accident. An event of abuse also comes up during the second sessions, and at the end of this session Sarah leaves with more pain and more distress. Not understanding Memory Reconsolidation at this point, I feel nervous about leaving Sarah with her resurfaced memories. Thankfully, she's back for her next session. After patiently addressing her emotions, she can retell the abuse trauma without an emotional charge. Sarah's pain decreases until on the fourth and fifth sessions she feels no pain from her fibromyalgia. I have not learned about Memory Reconsolidation at this point, but I feel thankful Sarah has reached a level of zero pain by doing the EFT tapping protocol with me.

Two years in the future Sarah will see me again, her pain having come back. By then I will have learned about Memory Reconsolidation and I will have created The ICE Method. We'll address different emotional issues that have surfaced since our first sessions, and her pain will return to zero.

As with Sarah's situation, like for most people, the emotions of memories usually appear to stay stuck permanently. When we recall an emotional molecule from an experience of years earlier, we begin creating more of the *same* emotional peptides. These peptides then cause a reaction in our body, which is why we go into fight/flight/freeze mode even years after a traumatic memory. In Sarah's case her pain symptoms felt immediately more severe. If a memory stored with fear, when you recall that memory you feel fear again.

According to what's currently known about brain science, you can only remove the fear or anger or sadness from a memory if you create new different peptides for reconsolidating the memory. If you don't change the available emotional peptide, then the old molecule of emotion reglues the memory with the same emotion.

This is what usually happens when we recall a fear or anger or sadness emotion - we react to that emotion, create more of it and store the memory with it again, over and over again. Most of us don't have Memory Reconsolidation as a part of our awareness. Most of us don't know how simple it is to transform our stored emotional upsets to a permanent calm state.

Transforming emotional storage.

In terms of Memory Reconsolidation, the emotions of memories can reconsolidate for something like four hours after the memory gets activated. You can think of this window as the time it takes for the emotional glue to set. When you activate a memory, you recall the emotion that the memory originally stored with. Then you have a window of time during which this set of brain cells is open to whatever new emotional peptide becomes available for storage. Without some type of intervention, the old emotion remains the only one available and the memory restabilizes without any change in emotion. This is most people's experience. This was James's experience of continuing to feel his fear of spiders through all the decades of his life. This had been Sarah's experience following her car accident.

In Nader and Schafe's original Memory Reconsolidation experiment,[22] they trained a fear memory into four mice. Later they exposed the mice to the fearful situation again and reactivated the fear memory. Then, just after the re-exposure, they injected the mice with anisomycin. This blocked the standard reconsolidation process so the fear peptides did not store when the memory reconsolidated. When the mice were later exposed to the test situation, they displayed no fear. In this way they discovered that emotions had to be reconsolidated after they had been activated. When they blocked reconsolidation with the anisomycin, the fear emotion no longer remained. Over 500 experiments have been conducted confirming and exploring the details of Memory Reconsolidation. Most of the tests have been done using laboratory animals, but a few studies have been done with humans.[23] Most testing has involved using chemical injections to block the reconsolidation of the original fear peptides.

When I first start reading about Memory Reconsolidation I am not thinking about injecting drugs into a mouse brain. My mind goes immediately to Candace Pert explaining how emotions create peptide chemicals that store in our synapses and also direct our mind and body. I am also thinking about EFT that I use daily, and all the emotional transformations that people experience when they use the tapping protocol.

3 – Paying Attention

"I don't know," I tell my neighbor, "but we can try."

My neighbor's brother has come to visit from Florida. Ten months ago he started suffering from a frozen right shoulder. As soon as he lifts it more than six inches from his side the pain feels excruciating.

Jeff comes over to my house and tells me he has already done x-ray tests, and also tried exercises and physical therapy. The therapy has helped a bit, but he can't raise his arm out to his side. I'm still using EFT at the time I meet with Jeff.

We start out with a first round of EFT that I use to show him the tapping pattern and get him used to the language. "Even though I have this shoulder pain, I deeply love and accept myself."

After this first round, he tests his range of motion, looking quizzical, skeptical and pleased, all at the same time. "It feels a little better," he says. "I can move it a few more inches before it hurts."

I have been reading about Memory Reconsolidation for a month now. I still use the EFT tapping method, but my focus has changed. I have my attention on what emotional peptides might have stored in the synapses of Jeff's brain that affect how his body works.

"If you think about your arm pain," I ask, "was anything different happening around the time your shoulder froze?"

"Lots actually," Jeff begins. "My wife lost her job, which means I picked up a second job. Plus about that time I was trying to get a new business started."

Jeff thinks a moment longer. "So, I've been really busy," he tells me, "but two of the couples we've been closest to for many years also separated about that same time and both ended up divorced. My wife and I have been supporting our friends this past year, but there's so much drama. I feel like we haven't had a moment to ourselves. I know I'm always tired. That's actually why we came to see my brother Nick, just to get away for a few days."

"If you think about this past year, what emotion do you feel? Is it anger, fear, sadness, or another emotion? Take a minute and see what shows up when you pay attention."

"I feel fear." Jeff tells me.

"And when you pay attention to that fear, do you feel it only in your shoulder, or do you sense it anywhere else?"

"Actually, my stomach just started feeling nauseous."

Jeff and I start some more rounds of EFT tapping. From now on we're paying attention to his stresses and his emotions. "Even though I feel this fear, I love and accept myself." "Even though I'm so busy and so tired, I love and accept myself." "Even though my best friends divorced, and I've been taking care of them all year, I love and accept myself."

As the rounds progress for the next ten or fifteen minutes, Jeff's frozen shoulder thaws. He can bring his arm straight out from his body without pain.

"This is really weird," Jeff says, "I'm glad I can move my arm, but how can my stressful year get stuck in my shoulder?"

"I used to think this was weird too, but now it actually seems pretty simple to me. Whenever an experience becomes a memory, we also store the emotion we felt during the event. These emotions store as peptide molecules in the synapses that connect our brain cells. These same molecules also instruct our body for how it should function.

"You've been storing lots of fear emotions, and probably sadness and anger emotions all year long. Those molecules have your body in a state of fight/flight/freeze, a state of constant stress. Your body is reacting to your wife losing her job, you getting a second job, starting your new business, your friends divorcing, and whatever else has been going on in your life."

"But why my shoulder?"

"I'm not sure, but I always like to ask the question of how my body might be trying to help me. In my view, the body always serves the mind. When the mind is calm, the body has a calm feeling. When the mind senses danger, the body reacts with fight/flight/freeze stress to protect you."

"I still don't see how that would show up in my shoulder?"

"I don't either, but sometimes it's a good question to play with. Are you right handed?"

"Yes."

"And it's your right shoulder that's frozen. Consider the possibility that you've been way overworked and overstressed this year. Having a frozen shoulder limits what you can do. Maybe your frozen shoulder is one way your body is helping you to not try and do even more."

"That sounds crazy," Jeff responds, and then reflects. "But it actually feels like it could be true."

"Let's try it out." We do a couple more rounds of tapping on the EFT acupressure points, with words like: "Even though my shoulder is carrying all the stress of this last year, I love and accept myself."

Following this Jeff can raise his arm even higher. It's above horizontal now. "This is so surprising to me," he says. "My arm feels so much better!"

"I know you've tried a lot of things to get your shoulder better, because it's been such a literal pain. For a lot of people, they feel angry or afraid or sad about what's not working right in their body. Getting better, for a lot of people, turns into a battle."

Jeff shares, "That's true for me – with all the things I have to do, and with all the problems this shoulder is causing me, I know I feel mad at it for not working."

"Right – that's really typical. So if you're producing angry emotions toward your shoulder, maybe it makes sense that it keeps hurting more instead of less. You're adding more stress chemistry to your body, instead of calm and healing.

"So, if you're up for it," I continue, "I invite you to thank your shoulder for trying to protect you. If you say words of thanks, you'll be creating different emotional chemistry instead of the anger you've been feeling toward your shoulder and your fear about all the stuff from the past year. If it feels okay, try repeating after me. It might feel strange to talk to a body part, but you'll be changing the instructional chemistry."

- *Hey shoulder –*
- *You've carried a lot of pain this last year –*
- *I had no idea you were just trying to help me out –*
- *I still don't get it, but I can see how it might be true –*
- *So I just want to thank you for your help –*
- *I see how much all this stress has been affecting me –*
- *Maybe you've been slowing me down so I don't blow a gasket –*

- *Sorry I've been so mad at you –*
- *Thanks for protecting me – I thank you –*

"Try raising your arm now," I invite Jeff.

He raises it to almost vertical.

"That's excellent," I say. "That's almost full range of motion."

"Yeah, and there's hardly any pain, just a little twinge."

"Fantastic."

Jeff starts to thank me for how much better he's feeling. It's been 45 minutes since we started paying attention to his shoulder.

"One last thing," I add. "If you think about this remaining pain, how much of it do you think you need to keep?"

"What do you mean?"

"Well, if the pain in your shoulder has been trying to protect you from having an overwork breakdown, what do you think this remaining bit of pain might be doing?"

"Is it a reminder to me?"

"Maybe, I know for some people I work with, it's easier to keep some of their symptoms instead of having them all go away. Do you feel like you need a reminder in your shoulder so you pace yourself?"

Jeff thinks about this. "Maybe I actually do. Whenever I have a lot going on in my life, I seem to just keep piling it on without taking care of myself."

"Let's try talking to your shoulder one more time. Try repeating my words."

- *Hey shoulder –*
- *I see how you've been protecting me –*
- *And I thank you for protecting me –*
- *Now I have this little bit of pain left –*
- *I'm wondering if I need it –*
- *Maybe we can make an arrangement –*
- *No pain as long as I'm taking care of us –*
- *But if I need a reminder, then you can let me know again –*
- *If that's okay with you shoulder –*
- *I'm ready to see if I can have no pain –*

I invite Jeff to try out his shoulder one more time.

Jeff raises his arm. Slowly he moves it through a rotation and finds he has full range of motion.

More than a year later Jeff comes back again for another visit with his brother. I see him in town for a few moments. "Everything is good," he tells me. "The pain never came back."

Even now as I write Jeff's story for this book, the engineer in my mind starts its old protest. And the rational skeptical engineer says, "This is nuts. Talking to your body. Tapping on your body. Telling yourself you love and accept yourself. An hour later recovering completely from a frozen shoulder. Nuts."

"You've come a long way," I remind myself as I hear this echo of my past.

When Jeff leaves after his session, my technical science side is screaming for attention. I have also just returned from three days of shadowing a fibromyalgia doctor. After her appointments she invited people to visit with me for a single session.

Maybe because I see these people one after the other, I start streamlining the EFT process. Get the emotion – get the person to a different emotional state – exchange peptides. I saw a dozen people on this first visit – all of them had improvements, a few dropped to zero pain during their session.

Engineers look for explanations, not for miracles. I wonder if the founder of EFT felt this way. Gary Craig was also an engineer. He'd been trained in a method called Thought Field Therapy (TFT).[24] TFT offered many specific acupressure locations to tap on, with many specific words to be used. I can imagine Craig the engineer trying to figure out where the effect actually came from. "What if you simplify all the different TFT possibilities into a single easy process? Whatever he thought, he condensed the process to a few basic steps, and it worked. EFT turned out simple enough that anyone could use it. People could also easily share and teach EFT, and soon lots of people started experiencing results.

"Why does this work?" I keep asking myself.

One morning soon after helping Jeff, I sit at home and play again with this question. I recognize something new to me. EFT is chemistry. EFT is Memory Reconsolidation of stored emotional peptides. And EFT is consciousness as well, the focusing of attention to change body chemistry.

EFT works. TFT works. A myriad of different methods provide results. My little shortened version of EFT worked when I didn't have much time at the fibromyalgia clinic. Candace Pert showed that emotions result in chemistry. Our emotions result from what we pay attention to.

- Our focus of attention creates chemistry. This chemistry signals the function of our mind and body – whether calm, joy, anger, fear, sadness, or whatever.
- Our attention can be captured not only by the present. Our attention can also be captured by the past or by scenarios in the future. The chemistry that controls our body in the present moment comes from whatever we pay attention to, whether past memory, future anticipation, or present moment.

As I follow this awareness a peaceful kind of giddiness arises. I sense a solution to my long-held question of why EFT works.

1. Whatever you pay attention to, you activate. (EFT does this by identifying the issue of concern.)
2. However you shift your attention from the activated issue to a different emotional state, you create new chemistry. (EFT does this by saying a verbal message while tapping on a pattern of acupressure points.)
3. When you shift your attention back to the activated issue, you replace the old stored emotional chemistry. You replace the old peptides with the new ones you created when you were in that different emotional state. (In EFT, this occurs by testing, by comparing what has changed from when the issue was first identified. EFT even uses a rating system from zero to ten so a person can rate the intensity and note the changes that come from using the tapping routine.)

Maybe, I think, you could use anything in Step Two that shifts your attention away from the issue. Maybe tapping is one way of shifting attention. Maybe that's the way prayer works – by shifting attention to a God focus. Or chants or meditations. If Steps One and Three surround this shift of attention, then maybe you have everything needed for Memory Reconsolidation to happen.

If attention creates chemistry for mind and body, as Candace Pert and others have shown in their research, then there would be many techniques to achieve Memory Reconsolidation.

At the fibromyalgia clinic where I'd visited I picked up a book called *Figuring Out Fibromyalgia*.[25] The author, Dr. Ginevra Liptan states rather boldy,

> **"Ultimately all the symptoms of fibromyalgia stem from abnormal activation of the fight-or-flight nervous system."**[26]

She then goes on to state even more forcefully, "Medical science has not yet figured out how to turn off the switch of the stress response that gets stuck in the ON position in fibromyalgia. When we do that we will have found a cure."[27]

Things are coming together.

- Mind and body chemistry arise from our emotions - which in turn come from what we pay attention to.
- If our fight/flight/freeze stress response gets stuck in the ON position, that happens because our conscious attention perceives danger somewhere in the past, present, or future.
- What could we pay attention to that would turn off fight/flight/freeze?

What if we could pay attention to "Nothing"?

Fight/flight/freeze turns on either for a real or a *perceived* threat. If we paid attention to *nothing*, then we would signal our mind and body that nothing in our outside world needs a reaction. If our attention could confirm no threat exists, then nothing would trigger our fight/flight/freeze stress response.

How can we pay attention to this nothing?

EFT gets you to pay attention to a tapping routine. This definitely shifts your attention and apparently satisfies the requirement for Memory Reconsolidation to happen. But what if you could help a person to really pay attention to *nothing*? You would have the perfect opposite image compared to perceiving danger and activating the fight/flight/freeze stress response.

One of the challenges to observing nothing is that many of us respond to stored trauma as if it is present right now. For many of us, long ago experiences cause ongoing stress in the present moment. Liptan again, "Studies estimate that more than half of women with fibromyalgia have experienced childhood sexual abuse…In one study, almost half of the male patients with combat-related PTSD met the diagnostic criteria for fibromyalgia."[28]

As I think about paying attention to nothing, I recognize I've never succeeded at meditation. I have a terrible time emptying my mind. I wonder if it's because I carry a lot of stress around that captures my attention? Millions of people meditate successfully, and thousands of ways exist to practice meditation, but I haven't found one that works for me.

As I think about a way to put my attention on nothing, I remember a book I once read. *The Secret of Instant Healing*.[29] Frank Kinslow developed a healing method he calls Quantum Entrainment. In this book he shares a few techniques from his decades of following Buddhist practices. There's one where you just let thoughts come and go in your mind, one after the other. As they come and go without you engaging them, their speed starts slowing down. After they slow down enough you can sense a space of nothing that begins to appear between the time that one thought goes and the next appears. As you simply keep observing, the space of nothing grows larger and larger and the thoughts become fewer and fewer.

I can hardly wait to get back to the fibromyalgia center and try out this new method. I've even had a name come to me, an acronym for the three parts of Memory Reconsolidation.

ICE   Identify – Calm – Exchange   The ICE Method

On this second trip to the fibromyalgia center the doctor has agreed she'll invite her patients to see me after her visits so I can do a study. Thirteen patients have both time and interest during the four days I stay at the clinic. Using the new ICE Method, seven out of the thirteen people who see me get their pain levels down to zero. Pain levels when they started had ranged from seven to a full ten out of ten.

The other six have either no change in their pain levels, or maybe it reduces one point on the ten point scale.

Thankfully, I find a clear difference between the patients who experience zero pain during their session and those who experience no relief. Everyone who experiences complete pain relief becomes aware of the calm space between their thoughts. For the six people who experience little or no change in their pain, none of them focuses their attention enough to become aware of the nothing space between their thoughts. These six people have such high levels of agitation and anxiety that they do not experience calm.

In Memory Reconsolidation terms, these six people living with sustained pain are unable to create alternative peptides to reglue their old synapses. Memory Reconsolidation does not occur for them.

For those who experience complete pain relief, they do gain an awareness of the space between their thoughts coming and going. They have an experience of *nothing*, and they create a corresponding peptide to match their mind body function to their external environment. Memory Reconsolidation uses this calm chemistry for replacing at the synaptic level, and people's body pain disappears.

By my next visit, I have settled on another method that Kinslow describes for getting to calm. Simply observe that between any two points you can become aware of a space that has *nothing* in it. By successively having a person focus their attention on first one point and then the next, their reactivity to the external world almost always decreases. When the reactivity decreases enough, a person can place their conscious attention on the space between points and have an actual experience of observing nothing in their external environment.

"It's like bringing down the voltage on a dimmer switch," I tell people. "The charge you feel is like putting your finger in a light socket. You can't go right from 110 volts to zero. But if you focus on one point that lowers the voltage a bit. And the second point you observe lowers the voltage some more. By that time you can observe the *nothing* place, the place with zero charge."

I see twenty-six more people during my next three visits to the clinic. With the new exercise for reaching calm, everyone feels it. Everyone who does the ICE Method and feels this awareness of calm gains significant pain reduction during their single session. Eighty percent of the people I meet with walk away feeling zero pain.

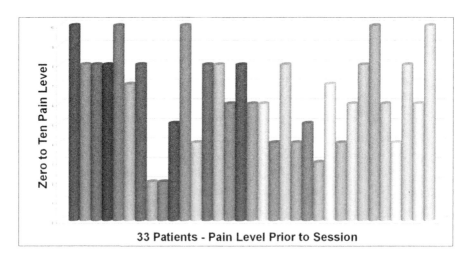
33 Patients - Pain Level Prior to Session

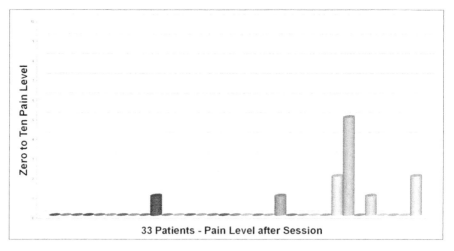
33 Patients - Pain Level after Session

This is The ICE Method. As you can see, I'm deeply beholden to the insights and developments of so many researchers, practitioners, storytellers and others. I feel that with this ICE Method I now have something to use, to develop and to share.

I still have some important issues to address in the remainder of this book. One is that most of these people had their pain return – and none of them came to see me for succeeding visits. Strange but true.

Before we get to the rest of the story, I want to write down The ICE Method process so you can have it to use for yourself and others.

4 – The ICE Method

As a repeat reminder to myself and to you, the contribution I feel I can offer is this:

- **I can share Memory Reconsolidation in a simple way.**
- **I can offer an easy-to-learn process for calming whatever upset emotions you have stored in your life.**

Here's the easy to learn process. You can use it without knowing any of the science that supports Memory Reconsolidation or any of the helpful details I share elsewhere in this book. Changing emotional memory really is this simple. It works for any situation, past, present or future that does not immediately and physically threaten you. (Immediate physical threat is really the only time you need your fight/flight/freeze stress turned on.)

The ICE Method
1. Identify
2. Calm
3. Exchange

Step 1 - Identify
When you consciously identify an emotionally-charged issue, you activate that memory so the emotional chemistry can change. When you *identify* an issue you look for any or all of the following. Don't do any extra work to analyze, confirm or deny whatever you identify. Without judgment, simply observe what arises in these three areas.

- **Memory** – See what experiences or events or memories arise when you pay attention to the issue you've identified. Don't dig – just observe whatever arises.
- **Emotion** – Notice what emotion or emotions arise as you pay attention to the issue you've identified. Look especially for anger,

fear or sadness. I always invite a person to be open to other emotions, but almost always, the core of an upset emotion holds anger, fear or sadness. Get as basic as possible. Annoyance is anger, right? So is irritation. Anxiety is fear. What you're looking for:

- ✓ Anger
- ✓ Fear
- ✓ Sadness

No matter what emotion people say they feel, it can almost always be boiled down to anger, fear or sadness. Not always, but almost always. For example, if a person identifies anxiety – the emotion of anxiety is fear. If a person identifies frustration – that's a polite word for anger.

Sometimes people identify an emotion of shame or guilt. What is the emotion of shame or guilt? Answer – it's different for different people. Ask yourself, "When I identify shame or guilt, what emotion do I feel?" Find out whether you feel angry, afraid, sad, or another emotion if you are identifying shame. Some people feel angry at the person who shamed them, others feel fear because of their shame and others are sad because of the effects shame has had on their life.

I've never had success helping people directly ICE shame as an emotion – but once they identify what emotion they feel about their shame, then the ICE'ing process can continue. We often talk about shame as an emotion – or guilt as an emotion. I have found that any emotion of anger, fear, or sadness can lie at the base of either shame or guilt. Find that emotion. Then continue to ICE.

There's no judgment in any of the emotions we feel. I'll say that again. It's critically important to recognize that you do not judge yourself for whatever emotion you feel. But it's also critically important that you identify this emotion you feel. Don't stuff away your emotion because you think maybe you're not supposed to feel that way. If you feel it you can ICE it. If you stuff it, the emotion will persist because you didn't reconsolidate it.

- **Body Sensation** – Let yourself feel the emotion you identified and see if you feel a sensation in your body somewhere, possibly your head, jaw, neck, shoulders, heart, chest, stomach, legs, skin, etc. The peptides you activate in your brain connect to peptides in your body – earlier in this book I shared this science from Candace

Pert's work. Mind and body connect, so identify whatever you feel. If you feel nothing in your body, no problem, but do make this check for body sensations. Way over 90% of people will feel a sensation in their body when they pay attention to an emotion. Not everyone, but by far most will. It sometimes happens that a person can't identify a particular emotion at the moment, but they feel a sensation in their body. Take whatever you get – it's all stored peptides – it's all ICE'able.

To use the ICE Method, the first step is what we just described; *identifying* your upset. You are checking for memories, for emotions, and for sensations in your body.

Step 2 - Calm

When you *identify* your issue, you will feel your reactivity – you just did that in the identify step of The ICE Method. A stored peptide chemistry corresponds to this reaction. Now we need to step outside of that reactivity. The *calm* step of ICE can occur in many ways, but the requirement is to get yourself out of the emotional reactivity you feel about what you identified. Focusing on two-points and empty-space between provides a simple way that works for most people. I'll provide some other ways of experiencing the calm state elsewhere in this book, including a way of feeling an energy "buzz" when we get to the chapter on quantum. For now, here's the two-point method.

- **Observe a single point**. Any point within your field of vision will work. The top of a tree, the corner of a picture frame, a dot in the pattern of an upholstered chair, a doorknob, whatever. Whatever you pay attention to with your mind will cause the chemistry of your body to follow.

    A moment ago when you identified your upset issue, your body chemistry and body function adjusted to support the emotion of what you identified. If you felt anger or fear, your body went into a state of fight/flight/freeze stress. Now observing this single point, you consciously focus on something simple, so the chemistry of your mind and body changes. Now your mind and body corresponds to this simpler state of reduced emotional charge. You may already even begin to feel a sense of relaxation. All because you made a conscious choice to observe a single point.

- **Observe a second point.** After a moment of observing the first point, shift your attention to a second point, not too far distant from the first. Repeat the same exact process. Again, you focus on something simple so your body chemistry continues to relax. If you imagine your stress response represents a certain voltage, then observing the first point reduces your body voltage somewhat, and the second point reduces your body voltage further.
- **Finally, observe the space between the two points.** Imagine this as empty space with nothing in it. You may have a wall or a mountain or the sky in the background of what you observe. No matter what you have in the background, imagine this empty space that exists directly between the two points out in front of the background. If you can *imagine* this empty space in your mind, then you can *observe* it with your mind. When you observe this empty space, you observe nothing. When you observe nothing in your outside world, your mind gets the message there is nothing to react to. When you observe this empty space you can imagine it has zero voltage – no charge.

Since your body chemistry always follows your mind, your fight/flight/freeze stress response turns off. You create peptides corresponding to this state of calm. Your body switches from reacting to the outside environment to focusing on only your internal environment. You switch from fight/flight/freeze to internal rest and restoration.[30]

Just getting to this state of rest and restoration will benefit you greatly. Living without your stress response turned on will give you better health. But you can do more. If you do all three steps of The ICE Method, then this peptide of calm can also transform the upset memory you identified a moment ago.

Step 3 - Exchange

Once you reach the calm state, observe your original upset again. Observe exactly the same things you identified as an upset; the memory, the emotion and the sensation in your body. You activated this in the first step. In this third step you now reconsolidate the old upset. All you need to do is to bring your conscious attention back to the original upset after you experience the calm space – then you will reconsolidate your old memory.

The process of Memory Reconsolidation, in chemical terms is this simple:

1. **Identify** - This activates the old chemistry
2. **Calm** - Observe a calm space – this creates new chemistry that carries the instruction of non-reactivity for your mind and body.
3. **Exchange** – When you do Step One and then Step Two, the old emotional chemistry stored in the synapse of the memory is ready to be replaced. Observe back on the old memory and the old upset chemistry is replaced with the new calm chemistry you generated in Step Two.

One important note – you need to observe back on exactly what you activated in the Identify step. You only activate what you consciously observe. Unactivated memories can't be reconsolidated until they are activated.

Yes, it really is this simple, this is the mechanism of Memory Reconsolidation in action. Follow the mechanism, and you can transform the stored emotion of any memory and render it permanently calm.

If you like to dance, or if you like as many visuals as possible, Memory Reconsolidation is also this three-step dance.

1. **Step In** – Step in and identify your issue
2. **Step Out** – Step out of the issue by observing a calm space
3. **Step Back In** – Exchange peptides when you observe again the issue you identified.

What you just did was a first round of ICE. What you reconsolidated was whatever you activated during the Identify step. When you go back to observe the exact thing you originally identified, you might find something new has shown up. For instance you might feel anger initially, and then when you look back you feel sadness. This happens because the anger reconsolidated, and now you are paying attention to the sadness. When you recognize this sadness, as an example, you begin activating additional memory and additional synapses. When this happens, and it happens more often than not, you can start another round of ICE.

Subsequent Rounds

When you exchange peptides, you will replace whatever synaptic connections you activated with the new peptides of calm. This is the science of the process.

After one round of ICE, you may feel completely calm. Or you might not feel calm – something new may have come into your awareness. New synapses activate when you experience a new memory or emotion or bodily sensation. This would make sense, given that life is complex and you have 80 billion brain cells and trillions of synaptic connections between these cells. ICE can reconsolidate whatever you activate. As long as you keep identifying new memories or emotions or bodily sensations, you can keep ICE'ing.

Repeat the ICE process with whatever shows up as not calm in your life, and your life will grow increasingly calm. If you like the image of the three dance steps, just keep stepping in and stepping out until the dance floor is calm. Later, if (or more likely *when*) the next upset arrives, do another round of the three-step dance.

I have people tell me they have so much stored stuff that they'll never get through it. Life can sure feel like that. But ICE offers a tool to take care of whatever upset shows up right now. Whether your pile of stuff feels large or small, ICE is really this simple, and it can be applied over and over again. Yes, you might have a lot of stuff, but would you rather take care of the emotional charges as they arise, or would you rather have them persist for the rest of your life?

Whatever you ICE becomes permanently calm. Perhaps a different way to look at overwhelming issues might be, "With such a big pile of upsets in my life, wouldn't it be awesome to have at least one of them become calm right now?" I will talk much more about this in Part Two – in fact I have a whole chapter on taking time to really know what you want. Knowing what you want makes a huge difference.

Introducing Part Two

Which brings me to the rest of this book. What I just showed you provides a simple method to deal with any particular upset, provided it does not immediately physically threaten your life.

In Part Two I will show you how to bring calm to large chunks of your life, including the patterns and reactivities you picked up as a child. These patterns have most likely been guiding your life ever since. You won't need to ICE every one of the million upsets in your life, you can address the pattern. Lots of our patterns serve us well, and we won't mess with those. But for many of us, we keep using the same childhood patterns that worked for us in our earliest years. We often get stuck doing the same thing over and over, even when we wish we could do things differently.

What else will you find in Part Two? Other than the actual ICE Method tools, the most important item throughout this book is for you to pay attention to what you truly *want*. ICE cannot answer this question for you. Your answer can change anytime – it can even change every day. Some people want material things. Some people want emotional things. Some people want relational or spiritual things.

ICE *can remove barriers* in the way
of getting what you want,
but ICE *does not create* what you want.

ICE can give you a free space so you can create what you want, but the result of ICE is this free space so you can create. ICE frees your life so you can pursue your goals, your wants, and even your purpose without running into your old barriers.

Some of us live with highly charged reactivity. I've worked with many people who have these strong reactivities, including people who freeze or dissociate when they remember certain situations. I'll share what I've learned from these experiences. I will include suggestions you can use to keep your attention focused while you do the three required steps of Memory Reconsolidation. If you can identify an issue, get to a calm space and then exchange peptides, you will replace upset emotions with calm emotions. If you can continue paying attention in this way, even the strongest reactivities such as abuse, PTSD and panic can reconsolidate to calm.

As the barriers and reactivities of your life drop away, new horizons open up. Although I'm a pastor and worked in the religious profession for many years, these horizons remained hidden to me until my life started transforming from reactivity to calm. The spiritual journey develops in lock step with our development of non-attachment in our life. While this can happen through following a religious tradition, it did not for me, even as a pastor in the Christian church. Reactivity creates roadblocks on the spiritual journey, and my reactivities never dissipated during my time in the church. Memory Reconsolidation allowed me to finally calm and begin transforming my life. As ICE removes your roadblocks, you may find that changing the stored peptides in your brain leads you towards greater awareness.

And finally, Part Two includes a look at integrating ICE with other methods and also a perspective from the quantum framework. Everything you learn in this book applies the understanding of chemistry stored at synapses in your brain. Once you identify that chemistry, you can replace it with different chemistry you create by a method of conscious awareness. ICE provides a simple way to do this, but as long as the three steps of Memory Reconsolidation happen, you'll experience emotional transformation. I want this discovery of Memory Reconsolidation to find the best and the broadest applications.

Part Two

Living The ICE Method

5 – Dad's Memory is Still Alive

"Lars, you can't leave people like this after you finish ICE'ing with them!" Penny sits in our living room, a friend of Anne's and mine from a nearby city. She's been with us on the entire ICE journey since I first became aware of Memory Reconsolidation.

"I'm a soggy puddle of tears these last three days. This morning I saw a little Facebook clip of a kitten licking a dog and I started crying all over again. I feel afraid to go in public. I have no control over when I start crying."

Six months earlier, Penny had done a couple ICE sessions with me after her mother died. When she came to complete calm about the difficult relationship she'd had with her mother, I suggested paying attention to her father. He had died many years earlier, but the reaction was immediate.

"No way. That stuff never comes back out." Until last week when Penny called and told me, "It's time, can you do some ICE with me about my dad? I feel like everything I think about doing with a new job or a relationship keeps bringing me up against my childhood."

We set up a time together, and the one session turns into three big sessions. In the beginning Penny can't get close to even having a thought about her dad without going into dissociation.

Dissociation happens when a person's fight/flight/freeze response triggers so strongly their body goes completely on guard and their brain function goes back to what people describe as reptile brain. Dissociation is the freeze part of fight/flight/freeze where brain and body shut down in complete overwhelm. In dissociation the person can no longer think or make cognitive choices. It's all about automatic survival. This is Penny, as soon as she walks through the door of my office, even before we sit down to start our first session. (In Chapter Eight I'll share more of what I've learned for working effectively with intense issues that continue triggering these enormous mind/body freeze reactions.)

"Penny, we're not even going to talk about your dad. We don't have to go there. I want you to put everything that charges you into a box, okay? Just put it in a box and close the box."

Penny closes her eyes. Body follows mind, and I just want Penny's mind on something other than her father. Whatever her mind is on, she'll start producing chemistry to match.

"Okay, what does this box look like to you?" Another question to get Penny's body to follow her mind to a different place.

"It's black, a big black ugly metal box."

"Okay. Go ahead and lock it up, chain it up, tie it up, do whatever it takes so you know everything is locked up in there, and it can't come out."

Her eyes remain closed. After a moment I ask, "How many locks did you put on the box?"

"Three."

"Do they feel big enough?"

"Yes, they're huge."

"This is your chance; want to add more locks or chains?"

Penny laughs. "Oh well, yes, let's put two more locks on that box." Hearing the laugh I know she has come back from dissociation.

We will have one long session each day for the next three days. I will use all my skills to keep Penny from dissociating back into frozen terror. We'll visualize a train where we can securely store the black box. I'll give Penny the train controller in her hand, and she'll back the train up around a mountain range, or sometimes across the continent until she can feel calm again. I'll use the two points and calm space sometimes. Other times I'll have her create a hot tub in her imagination that is full of calm. We look for calm places where she can create the calm peptides for reconsolidating these lifetime father memories.

I'm happy to admit I'm skilled at this work of helping people get to calm. But there is no mystery to what I do – it's all related to the simple point of this book. Reminder to self again:

- Share the scientific discovery of Memory Reconsolidation and the understanding of peptide molecules of emotion that direct mind and body.

- Share the simple ICE Method so people can reconsolidate stored emotional upsets.

While working with Penny, I count synapses. If I create a mental image for her to follow, I do it so she can feel the calm and create useful peptides with her consciousness. If I ask Penny to look back exactly on what she observed before, I ask so these activated synapses can reconsolidate with calm. And if I tenderly probe for new memories to arise, I do it to activate new synapses, start another round of ICE and reconsolidate more stored trauma to the chemistry of calm.

Synapse by synapse, all I do is help a person activate the peptides that carry the emotions of their memories. Then we take the attention outside of the memory to a calm space and create different peptides. Finally we observe back on the activated synapses and replace the upset with calm. Repeat.

We keep the black box locked. As the session progresses Penny finds she can stand closer to the black box and still remain calm. On the second day Penny has a memory arise that's not about her father. With dissociation never far away, I don't ask specifics. She agrees, though, to making a video of this experience in her mind.

"Start at the beginning of the video and just run it until you feel the first thing that's not calm."

"I'm already not calm, just thinking about the video!"

"Okay, back to your hot tub."

Back and forth, synapse by synapse, Penny reconsolidates this experience. At the end of the anger, the fear and the sadness, she calmly tells me that the experience happened in high school, her first dance, getting raped.

"You said this memory connected to something from your dad, that's why it came up a bit ago. Check that memory? Is that calm?"

"Not calm."

We go back and forth with The ICE Method. Soon she has reconsolidated this memory about her dad. Afterward, when she feels calm, I'll let her contemplate that some memory inside of that black box now feels calm without her ever having to open that black box. We've done enough for our second day.

On the third day, Penny ends up standing on an imagined seashore, calm waves coming in and then taking any agitation out to sea. In the sea, I tell her to imagine the upset peptides turning back into their basic amino acids. If these peptides return later, they come back as calm.

"Visualize the black box way down the beach, further away than you can even see."

After a moment I ask, "Are you still calm?"

"Yes."

"Let the black box come toward you a bit so you can just see something on the beach. Let it stay so far away you don't even know for sure if it's the black box."

"Okay, that's not calm."

"What emotion do you feel?"

"Fear."

"Where do you feel it?"

"In my stomach, and I feel cold again." She just did the identify step of reconsolidating this upset.

"Okay, send that black box far away down the beach again. And watch your waves of calm rolling in." Now she's doing the calm step.

"When you feel ready, bring that black box barely into view again, and see what you feel now."

"It feels calm."

"Little bit by little bit, ICE'ing as she goes, Penny brings that black box closer and closer until it sits directly next to her on the beach."

"It feels calm."

"I won't ask you to go into that black box, but I just want you to check whether the inside of that box is calm or something else right now."

Penny checks. Whatever she's going to find, she is not dissociating right now – she's thoughtfully exploring.

"It's not calm. I feel fear."

"Okay, back to the waves."

We do this a few more times, and then it's done.

"I feel calm now."

"Penny, that black box is right beside you. It's locked, but you checked inside it. And inside feels calm."

"Yes."

All this happened three days earlier. I'd asked Penny if she could go through some of those videos of what her father did to her now that the black box was calm."

"I don't want to do that."

"Do you feel a charge when you think about it?"

"No, I'm calm. I just don't want to do that."

Over the three days, I had learned that Penny had never gone back and re-experienced any of the abuse from her father. She'd always dissociated and frozen before she even got back into the memories. Year's earlier she'd done a ten-day silent retreat to try and work through the abuse from her father. In her thirties, she'd done extensive counseling. Even with all her efforts, she had not gotten free from the debilitating effects of her father's abuse.

I would have preferred going through a few of those memory videos, but this felt like enough. On the second day, Penny had even come to calm about one of her core beliefs – that she had done something to deserve the abuse from her father, and then because of the abuse, she had deserved the life she'd gotten.

Like I tell everyone, "Penny, you got whatever calm you got in these sessions. Whatever you reconsolidated will be permanently calm for the rest of your life. If something else shows up, it will be different synapses that hold different charges. If something does show up you can ICE that and come back to this place of calm."

Now, three days later, Penny tells me how she cries uncontrollably, an emotional basket case.

"Do you have a charge when you think of your Dad since the sessions?"

"No. He's been showing up in my dreams. But no charge. He just sits there. I don't feel any emotion when he appears."

Penny is a friend, and she's been supportive this whole journey of developing ICE, so I know I can speak more directly with her than I might with someone else going through a sensitive experience.

"Okay Penny, I get that you cried about cat videos on Facebook and that your emotions feel out of control. But," I pause, "didn't you get what you wanted from ICE, getting rid of all the emotional blocks about your father's abuse? You never thought that would happen in your lifetime. Whatever you tried before, all that stuff stayed stuck in your brain and your body. And now it's not."

I know Penny well enough, and I trust she'll give it back to me rather than shut down or try to start pretending anything but what she feels."

"Right, and that's amazing, and that's unbelievable, and it did happen, but now I'm an emotional basket case. I really can't go out in public. I feel like I could see a magazine in a checkout line and start crying right there in the grocery store."

"You said I can't leave people like this when I do ICE with them. So, what do you want?"

"I don't want to feel like *this*. I felt calm when we got that black box on the beach, but now I'm a wreck."

"Penny, I'm not going to say this to downplay where you're at right now or what you're feeling. I think though, that you're okay. I think this place is okay for you right now."

"It feels terrible."

"Yes, but you're calm about your dad. Here's what I think is happening. I see this with a lot of people who get through big stored issues using ICE. I think that once you get rid of the emotional upsets stored in your synapses you lose your old reference point. The abuse you suffered from your dad made you do everything you could to never have that happen again in your life. Your brain and body pick up your safe and dangerous settings during these early years. You just replaced those setting with calm. And that's both awesome and terrible at the same time."

Penny listens as I continue. "It's awesome that you got to calm, because now you can create whatever you want without being stuck in the old abuse. But it feels terrible because all those old automatic settings no longer apply – you have no reference point anymore. You really do get to create a new life now – but you have no more automatic history and no more automatic brain circuits to rely on – you're building from zero."

"It feels awful."

"All this crying," I ask, "It's new for you, isn't it?"

"Yeah, I told you I keep my emotions bottled up."

"That would make sense, it would have been really dangerous for you to express your emotions when you were getting abused as a kid. So that was one of your danger settings – *don't express emotion.*"

"And now I'm crying all the time."

"Right! It's not dangerous for you to cry anymore. But you don't have any practice at it either, so you cry when you see cats on Facebook. I think you're actually in a great place even though it feels awful. You're free from your father stuff, and you can start creating what you wish – instead of reacting to your father's abuse."

"I see that," Penny says. "But how long is this going to take? I can't keep crying all the time!"

"I don't know how long it will take, but you're building from zero, right? You probably want to stay gentle with yourself as this develops. Everyone has different settings of safe and dangerous. For some people it feels safe to show emotions. Their brain got set up for that. Yours didn't. So you have to create new brain circuitry for showing emotions. And you're now creating what you choose, not what you got stuck with from your childhood."

I call Penny every day for the next week. My wife Anne makes a point of driving over and visiting a couple times in the next days. Two weeks later, Penny visits again.

"I've been reconsolidating like crazy!" Penny tells me. "I imagined having a relationship with a man, and that set off all sorts of triggers. I was still calm about my dad, but all this stuff came up about relationships."

"How's the reconsolidating going?"

"It doesn't always come back to calm right away. It helped that you called me those first few days after our last visit. But everything that came up eventually turned to calm."

"That sounds great – you're getting really good at ICE."

"I even had some old mom stuff come up when I thought about jobs. I feel like I worked so hard to try and help her have some purpose in her life, but it doesn't feel like she ever found that for herself. So then I started thinking I might end up like her, and that sure triggered me!"

"What I wanted to tell you, Lars, is that I'm really excited about a job opportunity I found a few days ago. And I'm calm about it too. None of the old fears showing up"

Anne is with us; we chat for awhile as friends. Then Anne leaves, and I ask Penny if we can check on a couple of things for calm.

"Sure."

"I just wanted to check in on what came up about your mom. We haven't paid any attention to that for months."

"It feels calm right now."

"If you check back on that feeling of all the effort you put in to help your mom, do you feel calm about that?"

"Maybe a little angry."

Identify. Calm. Exchange peptides. Step In – Step Out – Step back in. Penny's done so much ICE that everything feels quick and natural. Back to calm.

"Can I ask one more question?"

"Of course."

"If you were feeling angry about the effort you put into your mom, how does it feel that you're putting all this work into creating your life now? Your mom didn't ultimately take what you offered. How do you feel about your own work for yourself?"

Penny has an immediate reaction. "Wow. That's a strong one. I guess I'm afraid if I couldn't make a difference for my mom, then all the work I'm doing for myself isn't going to make a difference for me either. That feels really strong."

"Don't worry. It's ICE'able."

After Penny reconsolidates these emotions to calm, I pour another cup of tea. "Two weeks ago you were saying I couldn't leave people with nothing after they finished ICE. Can I ask you about that some more?"

Penny agrees, so I continue, "What did you want from me two weeks ago when you were crying all the time."

"I didn't want to feel that empty. I felt so completely drained. I wanted something I could do or feel or be, instead of crying all the time."

"I didn't know you were going to end up crying all the time – but you sort of went for the everything part of your life, the abuse from your father that set up all the important danger settings for your life. That was your journey with ICE – each person has a different journey. When they do their reconsolidating, they get free from a lot of restrictive chemistry that stored in their brain and body. And then they have freedom to create whatever they want. What could I offer you besides that? I feel like anything more would be something I told you to add to your life - because I said for you to do it."

"I've thought about adding yoga or some personal development goals, or something like that. Personally I love QiGong, but I don't want to make that a requirement of ICE. I feel like any particular thing I add would be my personal take on what a person should create with their new-found freedom. And that would be me doing the work, instead of a person creating from their own freedom. I haven't found any way around that."

"Maybe that's it," Penny says, "Maybe what felt so hard was that I've never felt free from this in my life. And I totally didn't know how to deal with that."

I reply, "I haven't actually worked with anyone yet who has been free from their childhood reactivities, myself included."

"Really?"

"Before I started doing ICE for myself I had no idea how much reactivity I had stored in my synapses. I found a lot of anger in there! After I started doing ICE with others, it felt like everyone was running on stored peptides in their synapses. Almost everyone I've met seems a lot like you were, reacting to their stored peptides. If that doesn't somehow get reconsolidated it stays with them their whole life."

"I wouldn't have understood that at all until a few weeks ago. It still seems too crazy to believe, that we're so reactive to stored peptides."

"I know. And you're still doing that right now. You're just reacting to calm peptides. Which means you don't have the old blocks anymore – you can create what you want – and reconsolidate any new blocks as they come up."

Reminder to self: Again:

- Share the scientific discovery of Memory Reconsolidation and the understanding of peptide molecules of emotion that direct mind and body.

- Share the simple ICE Method so people can reconsolidate stored emotional upsets.

It turns out when you reconsolidate the stored emotion of a long-held memory, you really do bring those emotions to calm; permanently. The remainder of this book will offer you some deeper insights and experiences to help you use this neuroscience discovery in every aspect of your life. Penny's abuse from her father was intense, but when she reconsolidated the synapses in her brain and gained calm using ICE, it followed the same exact chemical process the EFT tapping procedure I had used years before with James and his fear of spiders.

As we continue you'll become more familiar with:

- The necessity of knowing what you want.
- Being effective when the memories feel very intense, such as abuse, trauma, and even PTSD.
- Getting to the deepest earliest patterns that set up your personal sense of what's safe and what's dangerous: what I call your *emotional Download*.
- Other scientific and spiritual perspectives that may deepen your appreciation for Memory Reconsolidation.
- Ways to think about Memory Reconsolidation so you can integrate it into other practices. The EFT tapping procedure is just one example of a method where Memory Reconsolidation creates results without explaining the peptide chemistry happening at the synaptic level.

6 – What Do You Really Want?

James knew he wanted to get rid of spiders. And he did.

Ben, whose story I shared in Chapter One, didn't ask me to get rid of his anger at his mom. This wasn't something he wanted, because he didn't even know he had that anger left inside. Ben and I were just visiting, and he was open to a demonstration.

What you *want* turns out be really significant. As long as you're not facing an immediate present physical danger, The ICE Method can remove emotional blocks standing in the way of what you want. With the blocks removed, you can get back on whatever path you want to pursue.

That little reminder to self keeps coming back - my purpose in writing this book.

I can show the scientific process of Memory Reconsolidation and the simple ICE Method Process so you can permanently remove stored emotional upsets.

With blocks removed, you can more freely pursue what you want. You need to provide the "what you want." This chapter will help you pay attention to the critical importance of being aware of what you really want.

This chapter also goes beyond the American cultural oversimplifications of "just think positive thoughts," "just work hard" or "just pull yourself up by your bootstraps." With The ICE Method you can have a technique for getting through your issues with more peace than most people experience.

Penny's friendship over these years of developing ICE allowed me to watch a person getting what she wants. When we first did EFT together, Penny had a migraine headache she wanted to get rid of. The migraine went away. The next summer big wildfires burned near her home, and she had breathing problems. She felt anxious about the smoke and her breathing problems. By that time I had just started using the new ICE Method, and I asked her for a moment to identify, calm, and exchange. Within ten minutes she could breathe clearly. The wildfires lasted for weeks that summer, and she had weeks on end with heavy smoke around her home, but Penny never had another breathing problem no matter how dense the smoke got.

When Penny's mother died, Penny knew she wanted to get past the upset emotions she carried. And when I invited her to do the same for her dad, Penny knew she did not want to address her father memories. Even though she'd had good experiences with EFT and with The ICE Method, what she wanted most of all was to stay away from her dad memories. Everything about the memories of her dad triggered dissociation for Penny, and at her deepest level she reacted against bringing up father memories. ICE'ing her father trauma was not what she *wanted*. Avoiding the trauma worked for another six months until every goal she wanted in life felt impossible because of the impacts of her father's abuse. When she finally came to me a half-year later, the old solution of avoiding dad memories no longer worked. She finally wanted to get rid of the trauma instead of continuing to try to run away from the memories. And with ICE, she got what she wanted.

I was slow to learn this lesson of *want*. Working with so many people, I know how simple it truly is to remove charged emotions from the synapses of our brains. The simplicity tricked me into thinking that everyone would want to use The ICE Method – who wouldn't want to make their emotional life constraints simply disappear?

With ICE, it turns out, you only get what you want, and if you don't hold onto that want, you're going to get whatever else you end up wanting more. I had an amazing experience with the group of people in the fibromyalgia study, but I did not learn the lesson of *want* for a long time.

Fibromyalgia Study

Put yourself in my shoes for a moment. Imagine you just helped 33 people in a row achieve pain relief for their fibromyalgia symptoms that had lasted for years or even decades. In fact, 80% of those people left their single session with zero pain. Pain relief was a goal they'd been pursuing for years or decades. And The ICE Method gave them the result they had put so much energy into achieving. I truly expected everyone would adopt "pain relief through calm" to be their new top goal. I expected they would make turning off fight/flight/freeze stress their first priority.

These were people who had been going to the doctor for years to get pain relief. When they finally achieved zero pain, wouldn't you have expected them to knock down my doors if the pain came back? After each session I invited that person to stay in touch, and to call if pain returned. I emailed and phoned each person after our session, inviting them to contact me as needed.

A few months later the doctor reported the patients were hurting again. No one from this group ever contacted me for more of The ICE Method.

Since I didn't get to talk to these people again, I can only say for sure that they wanted something else more than The ICE Method. My study and subsequent work with others clearly shows that The ICE Method works for delivering pain relief to people with fibromyalgia. These people searched for pain relief in a way that they wanted, through traditional medical care. Maybe they wanted traditional care as their first priority. Maybe they didn't want to entertain the emotional peptide basis to their health. Maybe they didn't want to be in a situation where no one had to take care of them anymore. Whatever they wanted, it wasn't ICE. If they had wanted ICE, they could have had it. I covered all my own expenses, and I didn't charge any fee at all for the people in this study.

In the time since my fibromyalgia study, I have watched people experience miraculous improvements in their emotional or physical health. Some people want The ICE Method as a tool for their journey and they keep coming back to it for removing blocks from their life. Other people do not. I have only recently grown comfortable with these realizations.

Whenever I have a session with a person I always tell them many times, "There's no judgment about whatever you feel."

For myself I eventually came to my own place of non-judgment about whether or not a person wants to use The ICE Method. Before I came to this place of calm, I had to ICE the peptides that triggered my self-doubt, as well as my peptides of anger, fear and sadness attached to my expectations of how others will act.

For me personally, I learned some powerful lessons from these results. I can work to create as great a tool as possible. The decision to pick up the tool lies in the hand of each person. Each life has many projects. Each toolbox holds many tools. When this all ICE'd to calm for me, I felt a wonderful peace. I still would love for every person on this planet to become aware of Memory Reconsolidation. I feel settled now to participate in this process without attachment to the outcomes.

Want

If you choose to use The ICE Method, you will need to want to focus your conscious attention back and forth between an issue and a space of calm. You'll need to actually want your issue to become calm. And it might turn out that you're giving up some positives when your upset issue goes to calm. If that happens, if you end up losing something during the process of gaining calm, you'll need to figure out what you really want most.

As I observe people, I sometimes notice how the initial experience of calm can actually upset a person. For some people calm feels devastatingly different from a person's normal stress. Calm disrupts their life. Calm can actually feel dangerous. Sometimes people let their fight/flight/freeze response turn on again, because they want that familiarity more than the unknown calm.

Others seem to find relief at an initial level, but the calming at the first level opens what feels like a Pandora's Box of unaddressed memories and emotions. Like Penny, some of these folks want anything other than opening that box.

And then I see the times when people discover The ICE Method and find themselves instantly and forever enchanted. Upset after upset resolves to calm until one gains a confidence that life can be calm now, and upsets can be addressed whenever they arise. These people want calm every moment of their life, and they ICE for every upset. This was my own experience. When I began my work I naively thought everyone else would have the same experience. Some wanted this. Others did not. What we want, when it comes to ICE, is what we get.

So, I ask you, what do you want? If you're like Penny, you'll find that your wants change with time – maybe even every day. If you wish,

The ICE Method can help you powerfully remove blocks in the way of you getting whatever you want.

A few examples: Take something as physical as wanting to double your income. If you have no emotional block in the way of this goal, then you can pursue it freely. But if you do have emotional blocks, then you have real barriers to doubling your salary. If you feel afraid to quit your current job, then you have a fear that blocks you from pursuing what you really want. If money was a charged issue when you were growing up as a kid, you might have an emotional block from childhood about making money. The ICE Method can remove your stored emotional blocks so that you can pursue your goal from a place of freedom. Once you experience this freedom you can see whether you want your original goal. Maybe that goal itself had an element of fear in it. Once the fear is ICE'd maybe what you want will stay the same or maybe it will change. Either way, you will free yourself from the emotional peptides that blocked your path.

Take something as spiritual as non-attachment. The ICE Method provides its perfect complement. Whenever you discover an attachment that stands in the way of your non-attachment, find the emotion, and ICE it back to calm. One less item stands between you and non-attachment. If you find something you *want* to stay attached to (like your house for instance), then what you want now (your house) has changed from what you used to want (non-attachment). As your life calms, you'll often discover changes in what feels important to you, and what you want.

If you want physical healing from a chronic illness, consider whether you are also open to the results of becoming pain free. At a workshop on improving performance one time I had lunch with a woman who'd been living with chronic pain for a dozen years. She was an accomplished healer using a number of different techniques. When I explained Memory Reconsolidation she could see how it explained results she observed with her own clients. We agreed to meet after class that day to try The ICE Method for her chronic pain. For the past dozen years the pain had been a steady level six out of ten. For all these years her joints had hurt, her neck had hurt, and she'd experienced a constant generalized pain.

"It's this easy?" Lynn asks. "Is this really all there is to it?" She talks more to herself than to me. I had just showed her how to get to the Download emotions she'd been living from since her earliest years. (Download emotions is our next chapter.)

Lynn already practices meditation, and ICE just adds the ordered steps of Identifying, Calming, and Exchanging Peptides. As she repeats rounds of ICE for the emotions and memories and sensations arising in her mind, each one goes to calm. Over the course of the 90-minute session her pain decreases and then disappears.

After the workshop I fly home. Two weeks later we exchange emails and Lynn tells me she has become a "full-time ICE'r. It's how I do my meditation now, and whenever anything comes up I ICE it."

Lynn's experience with ICE turns out to be a lot like mine – immediate enchantment. ICE somehow fits just what she wants, ICE grabs her and she grabs it. It happens like this sometimes.

"How's your pain level?" I email back.

"It's great" she answers. "Only about a two now, that's easy to live with."

I ask Lynn if she would like to Skype and do some ICE on the remaining pain.

The next day we meet online for a second session. After catching up about the workshop we'd attended together, I ask,

"Why do you think your pain is a level two now, instead of a zero, or instead of the level six you had before?

"I don't have any idea why the level is two."

We check out her Download emotions. I will share a whole chapter on what I call our Download, the emotions and experience and safe/dangerous settings we receive in our first six years when our brain wave state is absorbing our surroundings in a very special way. I'll share a bit about Lynn ICE'ing her Download when we get there.

Lynn turns out to be calm about her Download. Nothing new has turned up since our first session. If there had been upsets arising we would have attended to them and her pain probably would have come back to zero. Knowing her Download is calm, I continue:

"Consider that you lived with serious chronic pain for all these years. Do you think it might be easier to live with just a little bit of remaining pain than living with the zero pain you experienced at the last session?"

Lynn gives me an intense look.

"Would your life be different if you were a person with zero pain? Would your relationships maybe change? Would your responsibilities possibly be different? Would you have new opportunities?"

I let the question sit.

"Oh my God." Lynn breathes after a few moments. "I feel like everything would change. For my whole life, ever since I was a kid, if I didn't make things happen, I felt no one would even notice I was there."

Lynn wants zero pain. But even more deeply than zero pain, it turns out; she wants to be noticed – to not disappear. Her chronic pain for all these years has fit with her need to not disappear. Level two pain creates a perfect balance. The pain feels easy to bear at level two. And it provides enough pain so she can still meet her need to get noticed.

Secondary Gain

Getting noticed is one example of what people call a "secondary benefit" or "secondary gain." A secondary benefit often shows up as the good side of a bad situation. For many people, secondary benefit subconsciously drives a lot of our actions and our way of being.

Not everyone gains a fundamental insight into their life as quickly as Lynn does on this Skype session. She already has years of experience reflecting and meditating on her life. But if we open ourselves to considering secondary gain, many of us will feel some emotion, or a feeling in our body or we will have a memory arise.

For some of us, secondary gain holds tremendous power for our lives. Some people can't imagine life without this gain. For others the gain has such power it remains completely subconscious, controlling our behavior even though we have no awareness of this dynamic.

A personal example of secondary gain: I recently finished a phone call with a retired physical therapist. He had 40 years of experience helping people with fibromyalgia, long before the existence of an official diagnosis. His wife, a nurse, listened in on the conversation and offered occasional comments. I had called from my computer and I was slow to click the call closed when we said goodbye. Before he finished hanging up his phone I heard him say to his wife, "God that guy is smart."

Secondary gain. Smart has been a big deal for me all my life. I grew up imagining myself responsible for keeping things together in my family. Being smart helped me keep things under control. Control was the secondary gain of being smart.

When I switched from my previous job to pursuing EFT healing and then The ICE Method, I had lots of fear – stepping out into a new area where I was the newcomer. I had no smarts in this area, just a sense that a whole new world was here for me that I had never entertained before. I had no smarts, and I had little control. I wanted the new life, but I didn't want the lack of financial stability and the lack of a clear future. I remember one entire week of terror emotions. "If you go down this path, your life will never be the same." This happened in my early days of learning about EFT. I tapped on my acupressure points so much that week my fingers got sore.

As I opened to new possibilities and new uncertainties, I came up against all the fears that would have derailed me from my goal – except I had a tool that turned out to be extraordinarily powerful – I kept reconsolidating my emotional upsets, one by one as they arose in my path. Without Memory Reconsolidation I wouldn't have ended up near as calm about risking so much to pursue a new direction.

Without Memory Reconsolidation, would I still have made the jump into this new life? Possibly, but the underlying stress would have remained at a high level. Why? Because the stored peptides from my childhood will persist in my brain and body for my entire life – unless they somehow get reconsolidated. Think about this carefully, the vast majority of us on this planet live in reaction to our stored emotional peptides. In this oversimplified peptide way of looking at life we have two options.

- Follow our peptides: We can do whatever feels safest according to our peptides. We move *toward* whatever feels safe. We move *away* from whatever feels dangerous. If we're living with stored peptides, this happens mostly unconsciously. Without Memory Reconsolidation, this motion toward safety and away from danger is the best we can do to manage our stress.
- Override our peptides: If we really want something that feels dangerous, we can choose to override our peptides. Possible, yes – but overriding peptides will cause more stress, because our danger signals activate and our fight/flight/freeze stress response triggers.

As my journey progresses I have come up against more upsets and terrors along the way. But they arise less frequently, and they last a shorter time. Whatever shows up, I ICE.

I mentioned before how a person's wants can shift and change as they become more calm. That's the case for my own journey. In the beginning, I was fascinated with EFT but also very concerned about making a financially successful business. I had a lot of stored upset emotions around money, success and image in the eyes of others. As I pursued Memory Reconsolidation and creating a business, I ICE'd each upset as it arose.

As one of many examples, I worried about whether I'd be able to financially take care of my wife and my college-aged kids. By paying attention to each emotion as it arose, I transitioned from fear about securing the future, to a peaceful awareness that each family member can be responsible in this world. We don't know what the future will bring no matter how much money I accumulate. I grew peaceful with each of my own family members living our journeys without the illusion I can control our future. This calming made a huge difference for me – the person who imagined as a kid that I held responsibility for controlling the well-being of my childhood family. I had carried that belief into my adult life. If I hadn't paid attention and ICE'd when it came up, I would have carried those peptides and that way of being to my grave.

Public image also blocked me as I began developing Memory Reconsolidation. I had no awareness of how much it mattered for me to look good in the eyes of others until I found myself at home without the usual markers of success. I left a good-paying job to pursue this journey. The old job was fine, I enjoyed serving the customers and helping them with their questions, but I had no deep sense of life purpose in that job. The secondary gains, though, were wonderful. Money. Image. I'd helped start this part of the business where I worked, and it had become successful. I could easily explain my work to others. These were my secondary gains. When I started my new journey I found it embarrassing when people asked me how my day had gone or what I was doing.

"Writing," I'd answer.

Or, worse, "Reading."

Then when people didn't fill my appointment schedule right away, I found myself in the land of low image. The secondary gain of my previous job had been having a good image to project. I turned out to have *lots* to ICE before getting less attached to how I felt others were perceiving me. I'm sharing this bit about my own experience so you can see how much secondary gain can shape our lives.

With 80 billion brain cells and maybe 1,000 trillion synaptic connections in there, I expect I'll come up against more blocks in my life. Thanks to ICE I know I can calm whatever arises – if I *want* to. And if I don't choose to ICE my upsets, there's no judgment, I just get to keep living with the upsets as stored peptides in the synapses of my brain. With ICE, we get what we want.

Let's go back to Lynn and the secondary benefit of her chronic pain – a way to get noticed.

Lynne's need to be noticed feels so strong that she has reverted to a low level of chronic pain. When Lynn identifies her belief that she will disappear if she doesn't do the work of getting noticed, we start another round of ICE.

First we check for tigers. Everything that arises for Lynn is either memory from the past or fear of something happening in the future (disappearing). No actual tigers live in these memories of the past and anticipations of the future – no literal present physical threat. Disappearing *feels* like a tiger to her, until she stops and looks at her fear of disappearing. When she looks she realizes the issue of disappearing feels enormous, but a future threat of disappearing doesn't have a tiger in it. Confirming she doesn't face an immediate physical threat, she agrees to continue with ICE.

We ICE for her fundamental insight of disappearing, but we also look for particular parts of her life that fit the pattern; "if I don't make something happen in this setting, I will disappear." She feels charged when she pays attention to family relationships, partner, work, friends and goals.

So we ICE them and let Memory Reconsolidation bring calm to everything that wasn't calm. We attend to her particular situation and all the stored peptides she can activate and reconsolidate from long ago and recent past.

At the end of the session Lynn's level-two pain has returned to zero. We attended to a fundamental fear of disappearing that she'd lived with since her earliest years. A month later, checking in again by email, Lynn shares that her chronic pain level has stayed at zero.

What Do You Really Want?

"But I have this neck pain. I've ICE'd, but it's still a pretty constant low-level pain. I actually think it might be something structural in my body."

"How about another Skype session?" I write back.

When I share a session with someone I never know what the results will be when we address physical issues. Will it turn out to be "structural," or will it be "emotional" so we can have an effect? The question no longer makes sense to me in the same way. Body and mind no longer appear separately in my imagination.

I have helped people with stenosis to go from severe back pain to zero back pain. People with stenosis have a constriction of the channel that carries the nerves down the spine. Stenosis often feels highly painful. Same with bulging discs. Physically observable structural issues in the body, and yet the result of replacing stored peptides can lead to the disappearance of pain. I've worked with people who have shown me their x-rays, and their pain during an ICE Method session goes from high to zero. Not always. But often. I know when I help people experience Memory Reconsolidation, they can change out upset about their physical pain. My typical starting question is simply;

"When you pay attention to this pain, what emotion do you feel about living with this pain?"

In the face of this question, many people don't know how to answer. Having considered their pain as completely physical they have never consciously paid attention to what emotion they feel about the pain.

"Take your time," I offer.

In almost every case, a person will identify anger, fear, sadness or some other emotion about living with their pain. Those emotions are ICE'able.

As I write these words I am recovering from a skiing injury. Nine days ago I caught a tip while our family enjoyed a day of cross-country skiing. The accident yanked my body off the trail, and I fell into the brush. I felt my left hamstring pull like Saran wrap that gets stretched too hard and isn't going to return to its normal shape. Thankfully, we had almost returned to our car. By leaning on Anne's shoulder, I hobbled fifty yards and painfully lowered myself into the back seat.

Memory Reconsolidation Applied

As Anne drove us home I felt huge rushes of adrenaline going through my body. For once my fight/flight/freeze response had activated appropriately in response to a clear and present physical danger. As I've already shared, I ICE all the time - whenever I feel an upset. So I noticed that once I got back to the car I no longer had any present physical danger. I'd just been through a real physical danger, but now it was over.

I started going back and forth, identifying the sensations of fear in my body, then going out to calm in the sky ahead of the car, then bucketing calm peptides back into my body. I was breathing so deeply, blowing out fear and bringing in the emotional state of calm. I wasn't forcing myself to calm down. This was different. I was ICE'ing – paying attention to what was upset, then focusing my attention on a calm space with nothing in it, then exchanging the upset with this calm chemistry.

Because I'd done ICE as a way of life for a couple of years, I automatically *wanted* calm and not reactivity to the fear. And I got what I wanted – a calm and healing state, with the body back in a peptide state of rest, restoration and healing by the time we were home a half-hour later. I had taken the focus of my cells away from reacting to the fear of the fall. I'd refocused the cells on calm. This put each of my 100 trillion body cells in rest mode. Instead of my cells remaining tense about the painful fall, they turned to internal healing when I turned off my fight/flight/freeze stress response. As soon as this happened all my cells *automatically* began paying attention to whatever each of them could do to benefit my health and healing. Cells do this when in rest and restoration mode. I felt particularly thankful to know this on the day of my fall.

I spent the afternoon, lying on a couch, recalling the fall and seeing where I could find emotions of fear. I checked for anger at making the klutzy move on the trail that led to the fall. I checked for sadness. Every piece that I could reconsolidate away from fight/flight/freeze storage helped my body be in a state of rest, restoration, and healing.

Two mornings later, as I got out of bed, I was feeling really good. I felt so good that I came down the stairs without paying proper attention. My hamstring gave out on me, and I slipped and crashed down the last four steps to the floor. Whatever the first injury had been, this time my hamstring felt far worse.

What Do You Really Want?

I used the wall and got myself standing up. No breaks, but I could barely move my leg. A few inches at a time, I dragged it over to a sofa and carefully laid down. I start ICE'ing all over again – this time including my anger at being so stupid on the stairs! Two days later the back of my leg was black and blue from my hip joint to my knee.

As I reflect on this hamstring double episode, I realize that what I really wanted all during the experience was *calm*. A few years ago I wouldn't even know the difference calm can make. And because I had practiced a life of ICE for a couple of years I found myself wanting to get back to calm as soon as possible. I wanted my body in a healing state, and I wanted my mind calm in the face of all the "what if" and "if only" thoughts that arose as I hobbled back to health. And with ICE, once I confirmed I had no immediate physical threat to my life, I easily got the calm I wanted. Sure, I ended up with black and blue stretching from knee to hip because of the muscles that tore in my hamstring. Sure I couldn't lift my leg off the ground for two days. But I had calm, and I kept calm because I wanted my cells to be operating in that mode of internal rest, restoration and healing. A week later I took a hike – slow for sure – basically pain free – some stiffness. Did calm help? I think it did, right down to the cellular level of how my body did its healing.

Oddly, a week after falling on my skis, an excellent athlete shows up with a torn shoulder ligament. He is in the process of getting surgery lined up and doing all the MRI tests and everything possible so he can get back to his full potential.

I explain the value of having his cells in calm state rather than fight/flight/freeze. It makes sense to him. Observing for the first time the single point, second point, and the empty space with nothing in it, he tells me, "I've never felt this calm in my life before. Ever."

We ICE through everything that holds upset for him; the actual experience of the accident, the pain from the first day, the fear of the surgery, the anticipation of rehab, losing months of training as he recovers and the fear of whether he'll compete again at the same potential. We ICE all this to calm. More stuff might show up later. More stuff will almost certainly show up. That's life. If he *wants*, he can ICE whatever arises.

At the end of the session, he tells me how much this makes sense to him.

"You can live from this space of calm from now on," I tell him. "You'll encounter exceptions of course, but then you can ICE back to calm."

I ask him as he prepares to leave, "Is this calm something you want for your life?"

"Absolutely," he tells me.

If he wants it, he can have it. He'll go back to a world where few people know about the value of calm cells, and far fewer know about Memory Reconsolidation. Most of what he learned from life so far has been reacting to peptides and overcoming peptides. ICE offers an alternative. A very different alternative. If he wants it, calm can become the way he lives his life. Very simple. Also very different.

With all this talk about paying attention to what you *want*, I feel I should mention the increasingly popular process known as *manifesting*. People who manifest use their conscious attention to get what they want in life. I've been writing so much about getting to know what you want, I started thinking maybe this sounds the same as manifesting.

A few years ago I worked with a woman who had been hospitalized for severe depression. She lived on the East Coast and had been recommended by another person I'd worked with earlier. So we had our sessions by Skype.

As the first session progresses, she tells me how upset she feels. She had tried manifesting abundance in her life and ended up suicidal.

When I encourage her to simply let herself feel these upset emotions, she gives it a try.

"We can bring them to calm," I tell her, "once you identify the feelings. But we do need to activate the emotions and whatever memories and experiences arise."

I briefly explain the three steps for Memory Reconsolidation to happen; identifying, calming, and exchanging peptides.

"We don't have to stay in the emotions and we don't have to analyze them. We just need to let them activate so we can reconsolidate them."

"But I feel so scared when I do that. If I let my thoughts be negative, I'll manifest negative things in my life."

This woman has such a commitment to thinking only positive thoughts that she cannot grab onto The ICE Method. We try two sessions together, but since replacing her emotions of anger, fear, and sadness requires activating her stored experiences, she stops the process.

The ICE Method is similar and different from manifesting. It is also similar and different from the power of positive thinking, pulling yourself up by your bootstraps or almost any other process we might use to pursue a goal.

- The similarity? ICE and these other processes all have a clear goal, a want, something that has grabbed our energy and our attention.
- The difference? With ICE you directly replace stored upset emotions with calm right at the synapses in your brain. The other methods don't consciously help you replace peptides.

The other methods help you create new wiring and new possibilities in your brain. If you don't replace the upsets, though, you will continue reacting to your stored anger, fear and sadness. You will continue reacting no matter how positive you make your thoughts or how hard you pull on your bootstraps. I meet so many people who are like Ben, whose story I shared at the beginning of this book. These people tell me they've already worked through their childhood issues. For almost every one of them, if they tell me what emotion they felt toward a parent, they can still feel it in their body now if they check for it. When Ben remembered the anger toward his mother, he still felt the tightening of his stomach and neck.

All the work of manifesting, bootstrapping or traditional counseling can offer extremely useful and effective benefits. Memory Reconsolidation offers one additional benefit – the actual removal of the upset emotional peptides stored in our brain.

When I see Penny I often check with her about her emotions regarding her dad. Every time she tells me, "I feel calm."

The woman who was manifesting abundance ended up hospitalized for depression. I can't know what difference The ICE Method would have made for her if she'd engaged it. But we could have calmed whatever she did not feel calm about. She could have put her body into a state of restoration and healing instead of fight/flight/freeze stress. She could have kept on manifesting abundance in her life, but she would have been free of any emotional upset blocks that showed up as she pursued what she wanted.

Okay, this has been a fairly extended chapter on getting clear about what you want. Take your time on this – if you're still reading I assume it's because The ICE Method has at least pricked your attention. And perhaps it's already helped you gain calm about something you've carried as a charge for most of your life. As I promised you when sharing Lynn's experience in this chapter, we're turning next to The Download.

- The Download refers to the emotional setup we get during the first six-or-so years of our life. During these years our brain wave state is four-to-seven cycles per second, called theta brain wave frequency. It's basically a hypnotic state in which we receive the information that informs our sense of safe and dangerous for the rest of our life. We will live from our Download for our entire life - unless we reconsolidate the stored emotions from our Download.
- Whatever we have an emotion about stores as a peptide in a synapse in our brain. This holds true regardless of whether we can exactly recall the content of the memory, even very early memories. If we can feel it, we can reconsolidate it.

If you want freedom from any Download emotions of anger, fear and sadness, if this is what you *want*, then you have a literal life-changing experience ahead in this next chapter.

7 – ICE'ing the Download

My wife Anne and I ICE together a lot, often at the end of the day before we go to sleep. One night Anne says to me, "I just remembered a doll from when I was two years old."

"My mom made the doll for me. I remember hating that doll because she made it when she was hospitalized with her depression."

A little later Anne realizes the dates don't match – her mom had been hospitalized for depression when Anne was seven years old. But in her mind she received the doll when she was two.

I say to Anne, "I think maybe it doesn't matter how old you are or exactly when you got the doll. I think it's the emotion that matters, and you have lots of emotions about when your mom was in the hospital."

"I wonder how early a memory a person can have?" Anne asks as we finish that day and go to sleep.

Somewhere around four in the morning I awake with a string of thoughts.

1. What if specific memories really don't matter?
2. What if only the emotions matter?

A process I would come to call *ICE'ing the Download* begins falling into place.

- Ask the question: What emotion did my mom live out of when she wasn't calm: anger, fear, sadness, or another emotion? The actual objective truth doesn't matter – what matters is my *sense* of the emotion my mom lived from when she wasn't calm, my earliest sense of this.
- Then, take a moment to recall the emotion or emotions I felt as a child in *response* to my mom's emotions.
- See where in the body I feel this emotion. See if any memories, experiences, words spoken or even looks come to mind when I pay attention to my emotion and the feeling in my body.

- ICE this.
- Repeat for dad.
- Repeat for anyone else or any other experience that helped shape you during your early years up to six or eight years old.

I awake at four this morning, and without getting out of bed I spend more than two hours exploring my life with this new way of perceiving emotions for ICE'ing. I feel I gain more new insights and emotions during this single experience than almost any other time I can remember. I experience intense feelings in my body, shifting from stomach to heart to chest. My brain has very detailed sensations, one side or the other, front or back, feelings of pressure as well. All this as I activate the oldest stored peptides from the early years of my life. Even though I'm not sure of many details, the emotions keep rising with clarity. When Anne finally awakes sometime before seven, I am still exploring the emotions of my Download and ICE'ing everything that shows up.

"Your body feels hot," she says as she reaches over to me. "You feel all electric."

I tell her what I have been experiencing. Later that day we start ICE'ing Anne's Download. Soon I am trying it on friends; the results are deeper and quicker than any ICE or EFT I've ever done before.

Here's what I think takes place. This early age that I call the time of our Download holds a unique place in our life. Our waking brain wave state during the first six-or-so years of our life oscillates slower than during any of the rest of our waking life. At this age our brain operates at four to seven cycles per second. This is called the theta state, the same brain-wave speed as during hypnosis. At this brain wave speed we basically absorb our environment without reflection.

For most of us, in our growing up, we absorb everything that's going on around us, all the way from the useful to the abusive. And it locks into most of us for the remainder of our lives. This Download then sets our sense of what feels safe and what feels dangerous. Subconsciously, for the rest of our life, our compass is attracted to what feels safe. And we will do whatever we can to avoid whatever we picked up as dangerous. We begin living lives of "reactivity" instead of free choice. Watch a kid closely, and you can see the progression towards an established framework of reactivity that begins locking down around the age of six.

This powerful brain-wave understanding of our early years explains many things. Like why one person might be comfortable singing, acting or speaking in public, while the other person lives in fear of any public exposure. It can explain why one person might be more driven than another to earn and save money, while another feels safer when spending money. Some travel and fly easily – others struggle when they have to leave home. Theta wave state, back in those earliest years, locked down safe and dangerous for each one of us. If you take a class learning a challenging outdoor activity, watch the different rates at which people get comfortable with the new obstacle. Maybe its mountain biking and learning to do jumps. Some people take the class because they are "naturals." Others have signed up specifically to push themselves past fears they want to overcome. In a different situation the natural mountain biker might be the fearful one, and the formerly fearful person might be totally at ease. Safe and dangerous is an extremely powerful setting in our life that develops during the theta state of our first six-or-so years.

I mentioned in the last chapter that I'd get back to Lynn and share how she ICE'd her Download.

As with most people, I usually start out having a person ICE something specific in their life, such as an emotion they have about a physical pain or an anxiety that currently upsets them. This way a person gets to experience immediate feedback as they become calm. I do this enough times so a person starts experiencing how ICE delivers results in a predictable way. In The ICE Method workbook, which is published as a companion to this book, I show the exercises and the process of helping a person move from specific issues in their life to the more general aspects of their life and then to the Download they absorbed in their earliest years. If you want to do this work for yourself, the workbook will make your journey much easier.

For Lynn we had started out with the specific issue of her chronic pain. When she asked me, "Is this really all there is to it?" I sensed her trust rising for The ICE Method. Let's pick up her work there.

"Okay," I say, "you're right. It really is this simple. Everything we're doing is for replacing upset peptides with calm peptides. If you're up for it, I want to walk you through this thing I call ICE'ing the

Download." I explain what I've already written in this chapter about these memories we absorb during our first six-or-so years that form our life long sense of safe and dangerous.

"You're going to have a chance to bring calm to your sense of what feels safe and dangerous all the way to your earliest years. Is this something you actually want?"

Lynn says she does want this. I didn't use to ask and re-ask so much about what a person wants. But if a person doesn't really want the change, if secondary gain exists for keeping the charge or if a person has some other reason they don't really want the change, then those other charges will still be there after we use The ICE Method. And those emotionally-charged reasons will show up again in one way or another. In Lynn's case, you'll recall that her neck started hurting later, not the chronic pain from earlier, but something she worried might be structural rather than emotional. When we paid attention to this, she realized she hadn't been aware of her deep need to "not disappear." She hadn't been aware of how physical pain served this need. Once she became aware, and once she wanted calm for this situation, it ICE'd easily. Let's get back to the Download.

"Lynn, when you think about your dad, in the moments he wasn't living from calm, what emotion do you feel he lived from; anger, fear, sadness or something else?"

"Anger," Lynn replies. Sometimes it takes a person longer to identify this emotion, but Lynn's response comes immediately. For many people the awareness of our parent's upset emotion lives close to the surface.

"Okay, we're not going to do anything about your dad's emotion, and we're not even going to insist that you're right about this emotion. If I asked one of your siblings, they might say something different. All that matters is *your* sense of the emotion your father lived out of when he wasn't calm."

"Okay, now just pay attention for a moment. What emotion arises in *you* when you pay attention to your father's emotion of anger? What is *your* emotion in response to your father's emotion?"

This takes Lynn a little longer, but after a moment she replies, "I feel anger."

"Okay. And remember there's no judgment in any of this. All we're doing is accessing what's stored in our synapses. If we access it, we can bring it to calm. If we judge or deny these emotions, we don't access them, and they stay stuck forever, just like they've been stuck without change for all these years."

I ask the next question. "So, when you pay attention to your emotion of anger, do you feel this anywhere in your body?"

"In my head. And in my chest." Lynn says.

"Okay, your nerve endings have stored this emotion in these places in your body. Nerve cells are the same as brain cells, and nerve connections carry and store these same emotional peptides.

"Next thing I want you to do is the same as in any other round of ICE. See if any memories, experiences, words, or looks show up for you as you pay attention to your emotion of anger. We're not drilling down and analyzing these memories. We're just activating them by becoming aware of them. It's like going to a garage sale and walking through the sale, just looking without stopping to really deeply investigate any of the items at the sale. This identification of memories and experiences is all it takes to activate the synapses. When you activate the memories, you can reconsolidate them."

Lynn takes a moment to walk through the garage sale. After a moment I ask if anything showed up. Memories usually do arise, but sometimes they don't. If no specific memories arise you can work just with your identified emotional response, and/or what you feel in your body.

Lynne tells me, "Yes, I've got some memories."

We ICE in the same exact way for these oldest activated synapses of Lynn's life. After just the first round, she feels calm about the anger she felt a moment ago.

"You're reconsolidating stuff from before you even have concrete memories," I tell Lynn. "Take a check now about this anger and see what else might be showing up."

Lynn has more memories rising up and more feelings. After two more rounds of ICE, I ask her what emotion she feels about her dad now?

"Actually, I feel sympathy for him now. The anger is gone."

"Yes," I say, "That's true, the anger really is gone. In the chemistry of your body, on the level of the synapses of your brain, the anger is actually gone. If something else shows up, it just means it didn't get activated during this session. If you feel it activate later, you can ICE it to calm in the exact same way."

When Lynn ICE's the Download for her mom, she has a very distinct memory arise. She remembers being about nine. Her mom had gone on an overnight trip. Her dad was away on a business trip, and Lynn got left home alone. If it was a nine-year-old memory, it happened after Lynn's first six years of theta brain wave state. On its own, that memory probably wasn't part of Lynn's actual "safe and dangerous" Download. But Lynn said the memory was typical of the way she felt in her earliest years.

"Mom was always doing what she wanted – I felt like everything was always about her and never about me."

When she ICE's through her Download, Lynn reaches a place of calm about both her mother and her father. This calm goes far deeper than just *understanding* why her mom and dad might have been the way they were and done the things they did. Memory Reconsolidation actually removes whatever stored upset peptides got activated during her experience of ICE'ing the Download. If upsets show up in the future, it doesn't mean that ICE didn't work. Future upsets happen because synapses that didn't get activated during this session have become activated at a later time. Solution? Do ICE again on whatever has newly arisen.

An enormous difference exists between ICE'ing a specific event versus ICE'ing the Download.

- For a specific event, we replace emotional peptides in whatever set of brain cells and synapses are devoted to storing the specific memory.

ICE'ing specific events is effective, and it's great, but ICE'ing the Download takes care of much more brain real estate.

- When we activate the memories and emotions and body feelings that go back to the Download, we activate the core that shaped our actions and reactions to all the life events since our earliest years.

Eric finds me on the Internet. His wife Abby has finally been diagnosed with Chronic Fatigue Syndrome. For six months they have visited doctor after doctor for a host of symptoms: stomach pain, joint pain, muscle pain, dizziness, and constant weariness. From working as a leader at a small company, she'd lost so much function that some days she needed a shoulder to lean on just to get from the house to the car.

I tell Eric, as I tell every person I work with – I never know what the physical results will be. But I do know ICE can bring calm to present and past stored emotions. And when we do that, the signals to the body change, and physical health often improves. Abby decides to give ICE a try.

Our sessions take place online. I start as I always do, working with some specific upsets and explaining synapses and peptides along the way as we bring calm to one episode after another. When I feel Abby has gained some confidence with the science and the results of using The ICE Method, I introduce ICE'ing the Download on our second session.

Abby's mother emotions take a few rounds to ICE. The emotions of anger have many memories for Abby. Eventually she feels completely calm while paying attention to her original emotion of fear when she identified her mother's emotion of anger.

Abby's Download from her Dad ends up ICE'ing easier. She feels sadness in response to what she perceives as her father's emotion of living from fear. Memories arise. She feels them in her stomach. Soon all grows calm.

I get blindsided a moment later when I ask if Abby had any other important people who influenced her in those first six years when she put her Download together.

"My grandfather." Her voice catches.

Only these two words, but I see Abby's eye's change. Just the mention of her grandfather sends her body into an emotional and physical reaction.

"I still have nightmares that he's going to kill me in my sleep," she adds. She's already dissociating. Her body is in freeze mode. Her brain is in total defense mode; cognitive thoughts replaced by fear reactions.

When dissociation happens, we need help bringing our attention back. This is one reason it's useful to work with another person when you're ICE'ing or doing other personal work.

"Back to the calm space," I say to Abby. "Can you watch that single point?"

I ask her questions about the point she's chosen. I ask her to look at additional points and ask her to describe them. Bit by bit I help Abby get her attention off her grandfather and back into the present moment. The little points help her change focus. Other things might work as well – simple things, snagging her attention by focusing into the present moment.

By the time Abby comes back from dissociation, it feels like a good time to finish. We decide to meet the next day so she can continue her work.

The following session turns into 45 minutes of work. At the end of it Abbey has ICE'd the Download she received from her grandfather, and she feels calm in the presence of these memories that had caused dissociation the day before. She runs a video in her mind and stays calm.

We get to calm today because Abbey stays present and out of freeze mode. We do this in the same way as Penny experienced when she ICE'd the trauma of her father memories. Activating only the tiniest bits of memory and experience at a time, each piece gets ICE'd as it arises. As soon as any reactivity arises, we step back to calm. As with Penny's experience that I shared earlier, we make calm our home base. We venture out only to the merest hint of reactivity, and then come back to calm again. In my imagination we work almost synapse by synapse, transforming upset peptides to calm ones at the most controlled possible rate.

When I learned the Emotional Freedom Technique I was repeatedly warned about the seriousness of a person going into dissociation. When a person goes into this freeze mode, they risk retraumatizing the event and creating even more synapses filled with terror.

I completely agree about the gravity of dissociation, and what a danger it can be for people with PTSD, trauma, or abuse in their past. But the danger of dissociation is another reason I feel so thankful for understanding the chemistry of Memory Reconsolidation. When you know what's happening at the level of the synapse in the brain, you keep your focus on the peptides. If you can back off from activated peptides to a calm place, then you can reconsolidate stored emotions. The intensity doesn't matter. You just have to provide a setting where a person can step in, step out and step back in. If dissociation might happen, step lightly and activate only a few peptides at a time.

The power of your focus of attention makes all the difference. When you ICE a simple upset, you use your attention to activate a memory, step away from it and then focus back on it. Doing so switches out the agitated peptide with a calm one – permanently. When someone starts dissociating, you use focus of attention to divert your mind away from all those extreme peptides. Every bit of attention you can divert away from the trauma helps you change the body-mind instructions from dissociative freeze mode to re-engaging the present moment. Attention to a single point might help. Reminding a person of a calm image they previously created might help – maybe their calm house image, or gentle waves. When you help a person in dissociation, it's extremely useful to know that their focus of attention creates their body-mind chemistry. In the presence of dissociation I rarely feel anxious anymore. I simply start the process of looking for calm. I look for whatever way will connect with the person and start allowing their conscious attention to return to the present.

At the end of Abby's session she feels calm about her Download. If other pieces of it show up later, she can ICE them to calm.

For me, as a facilitator, I almost always focus on bringing emotions to calm and switching out peptides at the level of the synapse. Only rarely do I focus directly on physical pain levels. Abby's husband had come to me because of her chronic fatigue diagnosis. But we never focused on this during her sessions. Abby's pain actually went to zero very quickly during our first session, and it never returned. The pain reduction followed her becoming calm. Once we ICE'd her Download, I felt confident she could maintain her pain-free state. This makes simple sense to me – if her pain disappeared when her stress and trauma disappeared, then why should the pain need to return?

After our three sessions, we maintained contact for the next month. She emailed me every few days to let me know she continued living out of calm. She included whether or not any of her old chronic fatigue symptoms flared up. A couple of times she felt tired or had a stomach upset, but she thought she could ICE back to calm on her own. And she did.

Four months later I get a call from Abbey. She's been back to work for a while already. Things have gone well until this call.

"My pain is coming back." I can hear the fear in her voice.

"Last week it was just in my ankles, and I thought it might have been from walking more and getting more exercise. But then my knees started hurting again, too."

"Has anything changed in your life?"

"I've gotten a lot busier. I went back to full time again two months ago. That was fine, but now we've got a big project at work. I'm working overtime and taking work home on the weekends."

"How's the calm place going for you with things being so busy?"

"Well, that's the thing. I keep losing it and then I have to go and get it back again. Sometimes I feel stressed for quite a while before I remember to come back to calm."

"Let's get back to calm then. Get that image of your beach back in your mind, somewhere between your two points, and let me know when you're back to calm."

"Okay, I'm there," Abby tells me quickly.

"So, are there any tigers, any immediate physical threats in all this overtime work that you're doing?"

Abby hesitates, "Well…no."

"I get that work has put a lot of new pressure on you, but if there's no immediate physical danger, how is your body helping you by turning on your fight/flight/freeze stress response?"

"It's not helping at all, but it keeps turning on again, over and over."

"So it's perfect that you call me now. You're facing a bigger stress now than when we started ICE'ing four months ago. It's just time to figure out what you want again. You know that if you live from calm, you don't have pain. And you're experiencing now that if your body goes back to stress mode, your pain returns."

"Yes. I want calm. I don't want chronic fatigue to start up again."

Abby and I spend the next twenty minutes ICE'ing what she feels upset about. She feels anxious about not spending enough time with Eric. She has a growing anger toward her boss who could have planned better instead of ending up with high-pressure deadlines on three projects at once. And she realizes maybe she doesn't want to stay in this job, and she feels afraid about leaving her friends and finding other work.

"Abby," I say, "these are all big issues you just brought to calm. And they are still issues in your life. You're going to have to figure out your time with Eric, your relationship with your boss and your future job life. Nothing changed about those except that you turned off your fight/flight/freeze stress response and put your body back in rest mode. How do your knees and ankles feel now?"

"They don't hurt anymore."

"Great, you just got another experience of coming back to calm. And you know better than most how valuable that is for physical health. If you get out in stress mode again, you'll have to keep checking for tigers and then ICE'ing back to calm if you're not facing a physical danger. As your life gets busier and busier, you'll have to choose whether you want to live from calm or not. No matter how busy you are, as long as you're not in danger, you can choose calm and turn off your fight/flight/freeze response."

"I guess I know that. I just ended up overwhelmed."

"For sure, and that can happen to anyone. If you get stuck again just give me another call. Every time you come back to calm, you'll end up with more confidence in Memory Reconsolidation, and you get better and better at living with The ICE Method."

After I've helped a person ICE their Download, I'm even more confident they can remain pain free if they became pain free during their sessions. When we ICE the Download we bring calm to the formative emotional patterns of our life. When that becomes calm, then we can deal with whatever specific issues arise. On the other hand, if we start with specific issues but never ICE the Download, we never get to the core chemical emotional drivers that will keep coming up for a lifetime. Unless we reconsolidate our core safe and dangerous settings, these emotions will drive us for the rest of our life. ICE'ing the Download to calm is one of the most important adventures we can take on for the well-being of your life.

Now that you've gained some exposure and some examples about the Download, I want to shift for a moment from the actual process of replacing peptides. I want to step back and take a cultural look at this Download that each of us lives with.

I used to live in Nome, Alaska, as a pastor in a traditional Inupiat Eskimo culture. None of what I learned there will help you replace that upset peptide, but my experience did so much for growing my understanding of life. And I think sharing just a bit now, might help us think more deeply about our own Downloads. If this isn't your interest area, you can just skip ahead to the next chapter on working with PTSD and other extreme upsets.

The theta brain wave state we live from during our first six years makes good evolutionary sense, provided things go smoothly in these earliest years. At this age it makes sense for little kids to absorb their environment and fit into what exists around them. In tribal cultures back before agriculture, this worked better than it often does now. When small tribes raised children, the life-shaping influence came from a whole community. If problems existed in one part of a community, other parts might balance it out. The whole community participated in giving the content and emotion that formed a child's Download "handbook" for living the rest of their life. For hunter-gatherers with stable cultures, this worked great. By the age of six, when a child's brain waves sped up, the handbook had been passed on. From then on it might be edited, but a person's stored emotional peptides made changes difficult.

When I lived in Nome, a traditional meeting never officially started until the elders spoke. When they had spoken, then a younger person could add their thoughts. I didn't have the term at the time, but you could see the Download in operation across the entire community. Elders kept the traditions. Youth could speak, but only within the framework of what had existed for countless generations. Change could happen, but not easily. Change came slowly because the existing Download had proven successful for thousands and thousands of years. Yes, you can tinker with that Download, but you can't make a mess out of it.

On an individual level, the Download that each of us receives in these first six years resembles the elders in a traditional community. Received in a hypnotic state, this Download becomes the driving power in how we make our decisions. You know for yourself that you can choose to go against your personal Download, but it takes a lot of willpower, a lot of resolve. An example would be giving a speech in public when you feel frightened about talking to people you don't know. Possible – but not easy. Lots of fear stress happens because you manually override your Download, you go against your internal elders.

This theta wave Download state allowed hunting-gathering societies to live for hundreds and thousands of years, passing on their oral traditions and values from generation to generation. In our culture today, we live in the tradition of agriculture. We come from people who store food and gather surpluses. Over these past ten thousand years of agriculture, individuals and societies have developed powerful structures for who controls surpluses. Before the time of agriculture, societies passed stories on through oral tradition. The inventions of the written alphabet and mathematics allowed people to keep track of surpluses. Governments, corporations, economic systems, and whole societies grew to focus on exchanging surpluses while depending on a very few to provide our food. This built in characteristic of agricultural surpluses created amazing material progress, but also a problem of power.

I believe power and abuse issues cropped up in traditional cultures, but the overriding interdependence within each small community made *sharing* a top survival value. Individual distinction mattered much less. Ten thousand years of agriculture has turned this upside down. We still see sharing happen in our world, but the primary values, especially in our American culture, focus on individual achievement, individual acquisition, individual success and individual power to achieve these goals.

Individuality has some powerful upsides, but it can also have devastating downsides. Not always, but often, children end up suffering. These children grow up in hypnotic theta wave states – absorbing their Downloads, their handbooks for life. When abuse or trauma come as part of the Download, scars can form for life.

In our culture we have high numbers of people growing up in situations of abuse. I wish this didn't happen to children, growing up in these upsetting situations. When I served as a pastor, I didn't have any tools to help adults become calm about their early-life settings of safety and danger. I'm thankful I learned about Memory Reconsolidation. When our personal Downloads hold upsets, we now have a way to edit their emotional content to calm.

In this chapter on ICE'ing the Download, I hope you have realized that even the earliest events and experiences of our lives can be reconsolidated to calm. Now I want to turn in this chapter to an even earlier aspect of ICE'ing the Download; our time in the womb and our ancestors.

Consider that the fastest time of brain growth happens during the first nine months of our lives, the time we live in our mother's womb. All of these newly forming brain cells connect together with synaptic connections. If synapses connect, then where does the peptide glue come from?. Yes, from the environment around us, translated through the emotions of our mother. So our womb time Download includes our mother's reaction to her environment. Her environment will include whatever influences she has from father, work, friends, family or other emotional factors during pregnancy. This system ensures that a child comes "emotionally wired" for the best chance of fitting into the environment they will be born into.

Although we can't remember specific events and experiences from the womb, as I've said before, the stored emotions matter most. You can use a process similar to ICE'ing the Download for ICE'ing the time in your womb.

- Imagine what emotion or emotions your mother felt when she first learned you had been conceived and she was pregnant. We won't reconsolidate emotions of joy. But if you sense emotions of anger, fear, sadness, or the like, you can reconsolidate these.
- Do the same for the emotions you imagine your father felt when he learned you were conceived.
- Now notice what emotion you feel as you pay attention to this earliest time in your life. You won't have specific memories, but if you feel emotions about this time in your life, these emotions have stored as peptides molecules at synapses in your brain. If you have stored any emotions of anger, fear, or sadness, you can ICE these.
- So do this, in the same exact manner as before, ICE any upset emotions you may have become aware of about your time in the womb.

When I do this exercise with people, I tell them my picture of life starts with us having a birthright state of calm. Before we came to life, we didn't have any stored peptides. We came out of the energy of the universe, from what I like to call this birthright place of calm. In the same way, when we die, those stored peptides we carried through our life will dissolve into amino acids and we will return again to our birthright state of calm. I realize this is a belief statement rather than a scientific finding, but I find that most people can relate to this picture.

If we come from calm before our birth and return to calm after our death, I often wonder why we live most of our lives reacting to stored emotional peptides. I don't know the reason, but life does seem to follow this emotionally reactive pattern while we breathe here on earth. With ICE, though, we can bring our birthright calm into our experience of life, right now, before we reach the time of our last breath.

ICE whatever you feel emotion about during your time in the womb. When it feels calm, you can start watching a movie of your life from the very beginning – the first emotional awareness of your conception.. When you come to any scene, all the way from conception to the present moment, where you don't feel calm, then stop the movie. Whatever doesn't feel calm can be brought to calm. If you want you can now watch the entire movie of your life, and make it calm.

Of course, you should only do this if you actually want this calm to be the new basis of your life. In my experience few people have this life-calm as their experience of life. Most people I meet don't have any imagination that it could even be desired. But for those who want this deep sense of life-calm, The ICE Method offers a straightforward and predictable method for removing upset emotions from wherever they have been stuck in your life.

Two more brief points before we finish this chapter; ancestors and concepts. If you can ICE your time in the womb, is there any limit to what you can ICE? As I keep living with ICE, I find more and more things to reconsolidate.

After I ICE'd my Download, I wondered if I could use ICE on my parents' childhoods. I have some information about their childhoods. Both of them grew up on farms in Denmark. Both were young children there during the ravages of World War Two. Up until this time, I had only appreciated the *content* of what I knew about my mom and dad. With ICE I stopped to pay attention to what *emotions* I imagined my parents lived with as children. And then that next step of ICE'ing the Download, I let myself feel whatever emotion I sensed that I carried in response to the emotions I imagined of my parents. That did bring up emotions of anger, fear and sadness. I had never consciously been aware of these before. Since I could feel them, these emotions had stored at synapses of my brain, even though at an unconscious level. Once I activated these emotions, I got the same four-hour window to use Memory Reconsolidation and bring my ancestral history to calm.

How far back can you go? With both my parents being from Denmark, I'm a Viking, through and through. Although Denmark today often tops the list as the "happiest country on earth," the history of Vikings includes lots of conquest and savagery. I haven't finished ICE'ing all my emotions about my history, but I find it fruitful territory. When I have free time, I sometimes pay attention to what I know about the history of generations back, and then I pay attention to what emotions I could imagine those people living with. If I feel an emotion in response, I know I can ICE these feelings.

I'm not only a Viking, but also a member of the whole human race. There's really an unlimited arena for reflection if your mind likes traveling in these directions. And now rather than simply looking at the historical *content*, you can look at the history of the world for what *emotions* you have stored. Whatever shows up as an upset, you can ICE.

While world history might feel vague, I have an example that holds plenty of charge for most Americans – the political party of our affiliation. Political differences can hold highly-charged emotions. I've been subject to those emotions for most of my life. Over the years I grew more civil in my discourse, but it's just because I got more practice. Underneath the calm exterior, the same emotions lived on as they had for decades – my strong opinions about what is right and just and will make for a better world. In the world of politics. so many different ideas live with such vengeance.

One day I wondered if I could ICE my emotions about the opposition party that I knew was so wrongheaded! I paid attention to the emotions I felt, and I found anger, fear, sadness too. And they all turned out to be ICE'able! So I did. How do I know it worked? Though our nation seems to grow evermore polarized, for the first time in my life I feel calm about the parties and the politics of this nation. It doesn't mean I don't have opinions – I most certainly do. But I no longer carry a fight/flight/freeze charge in my body when I engage in a political discussion. I no longer have emotions of anger, fear or sadness toward those with different political views from my own.

I have something close to "scientific proof" of this. The impartial observer is my wife Anne. The experiment she has watched for all these years has been my father and me wrangling out our politically different opinions. Until I ICE'd my emotions about his party. Now I listen peacefully – not a made up civility, but an honest and calm appreciation that those with different political ideas operate out of frameworks that make sense to them. I must tell you, it feels much nicer now. Anne the observer through all these years agrees.

8 – PTSD, Panic, Abuse, and Extreme Upsets

Many of the neuroscience research papers on Memory Reconsolidation write about the *potential* application of Memory Reconsolidation to help people with Post Traumatic Stress Disorder (PTSD). Here's why:

1. Memory Reconsolidation can replace stored emotional peptides with calm peptides.
2. The intensity of the stored upset peptide does not matter. The process of replacement works independently of what peptide got stored from the past event.

I want to say this directly. Memory Reconsolidation, appropriately applied, currently is *already* helping people recover from their symptoms of PTSD. The Emotional Freedom Technique I started out with already has many published studies showing effectiveness helping people with PTSD.[31] I believe Memory Reconsolidation explains the brain dynamic happening in this EFT work as it does in The ICE Method.

Recovering completely from the symptoms of PTSD is a bold statement. I make it based on my experience with many people. I have the results of working with person after person who now lives with a calm they could not have imagined possible. I write this chapter to share these results with whoever it might benefit. I continue looking for places where I can do formal studies so Memory Reconsolidation can become a standard offering for those who suffer PTSD.

In fact, I write this part of the book today after my second session with a person who lived with PTSD since childhood. In our first session she flew into dissociation as quickly as I've seen anyone freeze. Her triggers activated and she reverted back to a full trauma reaction.

Memory Reconsolidation Applied

As soon as I notice dissociation, I switch all my attention to helping a person get back to the present moment. Starting back at the first session with Susan:

"Can you put all that stuff in a box?" I ask Susan. "You can make the box out of steel and put all the locks on it you want."

"There's no box big enough for this stuff." Her breath appears forced and fast, her eyes look fearful.

"How about putting it on a planet?" I ask. "A big planet far away, like Saturn or something?"

"That's not far enough away."

"How about a galaxy somewhere on the other side of the universe?"

Every little piece of content she pays attention to helps her bring her focus of attention back away from the trauma that triggered in her. Finally it's enough.

"That might work. We can try a galaxy."

"Try it." I invite her. "And make sure it's on the back side of the galaxy where we don't have to look at it. We don't ever have to look at it."

For the rest of the session, I stay acutely aware of keeping Susan in the present moment of the session. I explain more of The ICE Method, and I keep helping her stay in the calm space.

"Let's just do this calm thing," she jokes. "I like this space with nothing in it." We have switched to observing a calm space outside the window. When I'd tried inviting her to imagine a house as a way of getting to calm, she had reacted immediately.

"A house won't work. The house is part of the problem."

Back from her dissociation, Susan now calmly observes a space outside my office window. This gives the instructions to her mind and body to turn off her fight/flight/freeze stress response. Her stress response has been activated most of her life; turning it off now gives her a tremendously good feeling.

"You could live from this place for the rest of your life if you want," I tell Susan.

"I want that."

"You'd come up against some exceptions to calm, some things that triggered you into fight/flight/freeze. But as long as they're not immediate physical threats you can ICE yourself back to calm and then reconsolidate the upset."

"Yes, that would be great."

By the end of the session Susan has ICE'd a few very specific events, a relationship issue with a friend and an upset about some remodeling on her home.

We meet again four days later. Even with these very small items we ICE'd in the last session Susan tells me she's been feeling much calmer than normal.

"I feel a lot less attached to the drama when it starts happening around me. I used to get a heavy feeling when people started getting upset. These last days I find myself feeling; 'that's your stuff, not my stuff.' I do still care about these people, but for the first time I don't feel caught up in their emotions."

I made a promise to not bring the PTSD trauma back from the far side of the galaxy where Susan had banished it after she triggered in the last session. Before the session I had thought of trying something like what had worked for Penny, just gradually bringing that galaxy closer and closer and ICE'ing each little thing that came up. Instead, after checking in with Susan, I decide to try going right to ICE'ing Susan's Download. Staying cautious about dissociation, I start with her mother, not with her dad, since I knew he was the one who'd abused her.

Susan perceives that her mom lived out of fear and sadness when she wasn't living from calm. Next she identifies her own emotion of anger she feels in response to her mother's emotion of fear and sadness. She feels it in her stomach. I invite her to take a stroll through an imaginary garage sale that holds the contents of her life.

"See if anything catches your attention from your life experience as you notice the feeling in your stomach and your emotion of anger in response to the fear and sadness your mom lived from."

Susan chuckles, "What I'm remembering is yelling at my mother for months after she died!"

Susan ICE's her mom Download easily. When she feels all calm about her mother, I still don't want to mention her dad. I feel leery after her strong dissociation in the first session.

I tell Susan about my picture of before we come into this world, and when we move on from this world. I share how before our conception into this physical world, we can imagine calm existence as our birthright.

"I like that," Susan tells me.

"So, if you imagine yourself back in that birthright state, and then imagine moving toward the time of your conception, let me know what emotions arise."

"Yuk!" Susan exclaims almost immediately. "I feel nausea right away. I don't want to go there."

"What's the emotion?"

"The emotion is yuk."

"Anger, fear, sadness?"

"What's coming up are my ancestors – the women on my mom's side – none of them had a sense of self-worth. Can we ICE that?"

We can, and we do. She feels sadness when these ancestors arise in her awareness. After paying attention and calming what arises, Susan comes back to calm. I feel ready to try to ICE the Download she received from her father.

Susan already looks cautious when I tell her, "We're not going to return to all that stuff you put on the back side of that galaxy in your last session.

"All I want is for you to identify what emotion you feel your father lived out of when he wasn't in a calm space; anger, fear, sadness, or some other emotion."

"It was anger and fear." Susan's able to stay in the present.

"And what was your emotion in response to his anger and fear?"

"Fear," she tells me

I don't even ask for a location or any memories. We go straight out to her image of the calm garden she has grown so adept at accessing.

"Can you get back to the garden?" I ask.

"Yes, I'm back in the garden."

"Good, this garden is where everything happens. We'll stay here a bit. When you feel ready, you can check that emotion of fear and see what you observe. Then bring your attention right back to the garden."

After a few moments she says, "It's less."

"Where do you feel it in your body?"

"My chest tightens up."

PTSD, Panic, Abuse, and Extreme Upsets

"Back to your garden."

Susan still remains in the present, staying with the process. She does not trigger into dissociation. Many times people who ICE their Download do multiple rounds and go through many specific memories. When a person feels calm about their Download, I have them imagine a video of their life. I invite them to start rolling the camera from their birth or from their conception. In this session Susan surprises me by telling me directly about her biggest abuse experience.

"I was beaten so badly I spit blood up for a couple of days. My arm broke, and my nose got smashed."

Susan appears calm, but I ask her what emotion she feels right now.

She checks, almost with surprise and answers. "I'm calm. This is why I went to counseling for so many years. I used to tell my counselor to just remove this part of my brain. I didn't want it, and I didn't need it."

"Well you got rid of it today. You still have the memories, but the emotions have turned to calm."

"I tried all that counseling. I tried so many other things to get rid of those emotions. Nothing ever worked."

"You're calm now, but you should know that you might feel an upset in the future. If you do, it's because some part of your memories didn't activate now, and they might get activated later."

"I understand that."

"If that happens, you can ICE it back to calm. And what you did today, ICE'ing your Download, means you brought calm to a huge chunk of your brain real estate that carried this PTSD. Reconsolidating your Download allows you to feel calm in the presence of these memories today. And you can use the exact same process to ICE back to calm whenever you need to.

You have something like a quadrillion synapse connections in your brain, so don't be surprised if something else shows up in an agitated way. Just use this new tool you now have, and ICE it to calm. Go right to your calm place and then start reconsolidating. If you get stuck you can call me, and I'll help you through. If you want, you can have this calm for the rest of your life."

I can tell you story after story of people who no longer live with the symptoms of PTSD. Many times people need more sessions than what Susan experienced, but the process always goes the same way – Identify, Calm, Exchange peptides. When you use The ICE Method to apply Memory Reconsolidation, you always look for the upset emotions that have glued as peptides into the synapses of traumatic memories.

ICE'ing for PTSD follows the same exact process as reconsolidating memories for any other type of memory – with one warning.

You have to keep out of dissociation.

If you or a person you are helping dissociates, you have to get out of dissociation before you can continue.

Keeping a person from dissociating takes far more skill than assisting a person to apply the ICE Method. The ICE Method, as you've become aware by now, is simple and direct. Dissociation, on the other hand, poses a lurking threat that can sometimes trigger with barely a warning.

People with PTSD end up with enormous parts of their brain real estate dedicated to keeping them from ever again ending up in the old trauma. The body and mind, consciously and subconsciously, have created hair trigger settings to activate at the slightest possibility of the traumatizing event recurring. That hair trigger causes a high stress which takes a large physical and emotional toll.

PTSD and dissociation are a huge deal. The threat of dissociation and retraumatization are why some people with PTSD never seek treatment. It takes a skilled facilitator to help a person stay present and not dissociate – but these skilled people do exist. Counselors, therapists, nurses, pastors and others have the skills to gracefully help people stay present and not dissociate. If someone can help moderate the dissociation and keep a person present, the application of ICE is the simplest part of the process.

When I work with highly charged synapses, I remind myself and I tell the person I'm working with, "We're going to take this synapse by synapse." We're not out to activate more than the barest amount of experience or emotion or bodily sensation at a time. The less we can activate, the better. Whatever we get can be ICE'd, and then that little bit has become permanently calm.

Two things happen when you take this synapse-by-synapse approach. First, you actually make a bit more of the brain calm each time you reconsolidate a synapse. Second, each time you do a round of ICE, the person gains one more experience of this process delivering the results of calm. As the rounds add up and as calm builds up, confidence increases and the pace of reconsolidation usually accelerates.

The first time I became aware of working with PTSD, the woman made no mention of it. All I noticed was her frantic, glazed look of dissociation:

Ellen spirals right through the anxiety ceiling. Before my eyes her face changes color, and she begins to tremble.

"Whatever this is," I say, "it must be like a big mountain in your life. We're not going in there."

"Back to the calm space," I invite this woman. I walk across the room and stand next to the light switch. Physically pointing at the switch and drawing her attention to it, I tell her, "Just observe this switch. Just look at it for a second." She trembles, but manages to put her gaze on the light switch.

"Good. That's real good."

"Next look at this door handle," I continue. Slowly, she begins returning from her dissociated state. "Now look at the space that's in between the door handle and the light switch. Look at this space that has nothing in it. After a bit she can talk to me again.

"Listen," I said, following a hunch that is growing inside me. "You've got intense emotions stored here, but every emotion is made out of a peptide. I know we can replace the peptides."

"Don't do this yet," I instruct her, explaining a process that has just occurred to me. "In a minute, when you're ready, I'm going to invite you to stick your hand up against that same part of the mountain you just reacted to. When you do that, as soon as you get any emotion, memory or feeling in your body, I want you to snap your hand back away from that mountain, okay?"

She gives me a nervous nod.

"Just for a second. Then bring your hand right back with whatever you get. Okay, when you're ready, go ahead."

Cautiously she lifts her hand; then snaps it back almost instantly.

"Okay." I don't ask any questions about what she felt. "Now back to the calm space." I walk her through the two points and then into the space so she once again observes the space with nothing in it.

"Was it the same or different when you put your hand up against the mountain?"

"It was different this time."

"All right then. In a minute I'm going to invite you to put your hand up against the exact thing you noticed on the mountain last time. Not the whole mountain, just that one single thing you noticed last time. And when you do, as soon as you feel any emotion, or memory, or feeling in your body, snap your hand back to your side, got it?"

"Yes."

"Okay, whenever you're ready."

Her hand goes out to probe what she'd felt before and then quickly she brings it back."

Out to the calm space. Back to the last observed place on the mountain. Get the next impression. We do the ICE Method in this highly controlled way, preventing the emotions from elevating by taking just the tiniest bits at a time. We go back and forth six or seven times. Each time she snaps her hand back intensely, noting that she's gotten something more.

I haven't asked a single question of her feelings to this point, but finally I want to know, "You're still feeling things on the mountain?"

"Yes," she answered.

"Are they still as intense?"

"No...I can hardly feel anything anymore."

What a revelation! Here was a woman who just moments before was headed toward full-blown panic and dissociation from a stored memory. In the space of fifteen minutes she came back to calm and could once again engage the situation. Furthermore, she reconsolidated some specific intense past experiences, eliminating the charges on each memory that had come into her awareness.

PTSD, Panic, Abuse, and Extreme Upsets

In later sessions with other people with PTSD, I have used this image of a mountain and had people use their hand as a probe. It has worked great for many people. In the example I shared earlier regarding Penny's PTSD from her father, the mountain image didn't hold her attention. That's when I tried having her put the events in a box, and load them on a train. When I gave Penny an imaginary train controller she found it worked better than using her hand to probe her PTSD.

Whatever image ends up working for a person, the whole point is to help them keep from dissociating so they can stay present and ICE their trauma emotions to calm. If you can keep a person from dissociating then you're back to the very simple process of identifying, calming and exchanging peptides.

The acronym PTSD seems to be growing in use. I often hear people saying casually how they have PTSD about this or that. You will want to look at more resources for fuller details about PTSD, but I want to write a few words here that may help explain why Memory Reconsolidation and The ICE Method can help eliminate the emotional charge surrounding PTSD experiences.

The American Psychiatric Association maintains that a diagnosis of PTSD requires a person be exposed to "death, threatened death, actual or serious injury, or actual or threatened sexual violence."

The US Government's National Institute of Mental Health describes PTSD a little more broadly: "PTSD develops after a terrifying ordeal that involved physical harm or the threat of physical harm. The person who develops PTSD may have been the one who was harmed, the harm may have happened to a loved one, or the person may have witnessed a harmful event that happened to loved ones or strangers."[32]

Psychiatric researcher Dorthe Berntson co-authored a paper in 2008 "evaluating basic assumptions underlying PTSD Diagnosis."[33] Berntson and colleagues argued that what matters for PTSD is *the memory about the event*, not the event itself. And this memory can cause PTSD symptoms whether or not the event was life threatening.

**It was the memory – not the event –
that made the difference.**

I hope you see the connection to The ICE Method. Memory Reconsolidation works on the stored emotional peptides that are part of all memories including PTSD memories.

In 2012 a landmark study of 746 Danish soldiers was published. It was the first research into soldiers *before* they went to war. Before the soldiers went to Afghanistan, researchers catalogued their early life experience. They found three basic response patterns to the war.[34,35,36]

1. Ninety-five percent of the Danish soldiers did not suffer PTSD upon their return from Afghanistan. To a greater degree, members of this group had safer and more secure childhood experiences.
2. Five percent of the soldiers in the study developed PTSD upon their return from Afghanistan. To a greater degree, members of this group had suffered more traumatic childhood experiences. The researchers found two patterns within this group.
    a. The first part of this PTSD group had functioned normally before their war experience. Only after returning from Afghanistan did they develop PTSD.
    b. The second part of this PTSD group had the most severe early-childhood trauma. They already had PTSD symptoms before they went to Afghanistan. In Afghanistan their symptoms improved. They actually functioned better in war than at home in Denmark. When they returned home their PTSD symptoms again worsened. The researchers theorized that for this group of soldiers, being in the military provided a more stable and supportive environment than their daily life back home.

By studying soldiers before their war experience, researchers gained data that supports the importance of early childhood trauma for developing wartime PTSD. Early-life trauma can set a person up to view the world as "not safe;" as "always potentially dangerous." It makes sense that for many of these people their fight/flight/freeze stress response would be stuck on. This takes energy from the body – taking the body's resources away from maintaining health. Instead, the body's energy resources protect against the possibility of external threats. If a person gets set up like this because of trauma in their earliest years, you can imagine that later trauma might have a bigger impact for this person.

PTSD, Panic, Abuse, and Extreme Upsets

The later traumatic event *confirms* what the person already believes the world is like, and that this type of trauma can happen in the world at any time. The fight/flight/freeze stress response gets set even more strongly.

If the fight/flight/freeze stress response turns on all the time, that constant stress also wears the body down. When the body wears down it often eventually starts to hurt. Stomach, muscle, joint, head, and other pains become common. I gained a lot of experience in this area working with people with fibromyalgia and writing *Fibromyalgia Relief*.[37]

The good news is that when people use The ICE Method to turn off their stress response, chronic symptoms often start to diminish. The other good news, of course, is that the emotions from PTSD events can be brought to a permanent state of calm.

The takeaway here – the intensity of the emotional peptide does not make a difference in the mechanical process of Memory Reconsolidation. The intensity does affect how quickly a person dissociates. Find a way to keep a person from dissociating and keep them engaged in The ICE Method. Stay engaged in ICE, and a person's emotional trauma can transform to a permanent state of calm. Provided a person really *wants* this calm for their life, the process comes down to identifying, calming and exchanging peptides.

A person I once worked with for panic attacks wrote me some weeks later about another issue - numbers. Everything about numbers and math had bothered him since childhood. He'd previously used ICE to calm panic attacks that also had been with him since his earliest years. He found himself instantly enchanted with ICE and started using it for all aspects of his life. When we got together for an online session, he told me that whenever he had to do something with numbers, he would freeze, and he could not think. Dissociation.

In Jeff's daily work he helped schedule patients for therapy treatments. Just organizing the list of which patient would go first, second or third surfaced his panic. Physically, in these situations, he often felt his legs go numb. His body felt like it froze in place with no place to run.

"Are there any memories?" I ask him when we have our online session. "Anything come up when you think about numbers?"

"Yes," he answers right away. "When I was in first grade I couldn't get a math problem one day in class. The teacher made me stay after, and I remember feeling terrified. I just froze and couldn't talk or anything."

"Alright" I interrupt Jeff, "let's just go out to the calm space right away. This is a big memory." I interrupt only because I want to stop him from activating any more synapses. He has already activated some peptides just with the memory he recalled. As quickly as possible I want to get him out of numbers trauma focus and back to calm state focus.

Since becoming aware of ICE, Jeff has taken it on full time. A week after the workshop where we'd met, he had emailed to thank me with the words, "I have been looking for this for a *long* time." A few weeks later we met online for our first session.

Now I explain the mountain image to him, and he agrees to try it out. "When you're ready," I invite him, "put your hand up against that first-grade experience, and take the first thing you become aware of."

"It's the feeling of being frozen and the picture of him yelling at me."

Back immediately to the calm space. When he checks the mountain again, he has the feeling of being completely alone; all the other kids had gone home from school.

Back again to the calm space. Next time he checks the mountain, the images already feel less distinct and more fuzzy.

"Anything else showing up when you check the mountain?" I ask him.

"Not really. It feels calm."

"Okay, imagine being back in your work situation, organizing the schedule of patients. What shows up?"

"That feels calm too."

Sometimes sessions go for an hour or more, reconsolidating one issue after another; the emotions, physical sensations and memories that arise. In this case, just a few moments of reconsolidating the stored emotions of a first-grade disaster healed a lifetime of numbers anxiety. This man didn't have a genetic problem with math or any sort of a math handicap. He had stored peptides that triggered his freeze response whenever he saw numbers. From that freeze response his

PTSD, Panic, Abuse, and Extreme Upsets

body turned to literal survival mode. In that state, he had no brain capacity left for adding even simple numbers.

I tell Jeff, "Your response to your first-grade teacher was a good survival response back when this event happened. Freeze was the only option that made sense. If you'd fled your teacher you would have ended up in even worse trouble. Or if you'd fought your teacher, that would have been really bad. Your body froze, and you survived."

"Since it worked that one time," I continue, "your mind and body picked that up as a solution from then on. Whenever you faced numbers after that, you froze. It turned out to be a solution with unwanted side effects, like not being able to schedule patients without going into panic mode."

"This makes so much sense."

"Yes, and now that you reconsolidated that first-grade experience; your body shouldn't get activated by numbers anymore. If it does, it just means you have other triggers. If you do, you can reconsolidate those the same way."

Two months later, I check in with this man to see how he is doing with numbers. He emails back to me:

> Now when I schedule patients, I can do it without panic attack: The biggest thing is that my brain does not shut down and go into la la land. That is quite a significant improvement, I'll tell you!

Another month later I was back online with Jeff. He'd been ICE'ing constantly and told me there were a couple things he couldn't get to the root of. He'd told me that he'd had a difficult childhood, but until after we ICE'd his Download I had no idea of the level of abuse and terror he'd lived through in his growing up years.

If you think back to Jeff's traumatizing experience with his math teacher, it matches what the Danish researchers found in their solder study. Based on all the trauma he experienced at home, the traumatic experience at school served as confirmation that you always need to be ready for danger. Since the content surrounding the emotion was math, Jeff triggered on math for the rest of his life. PTSD. Until he ICE'd it to calm.

For many kids, getting yelled at by a teacher is just a bad memory not a PTSD trigger for the rest of their life. For Jeff, the math trauma confirmed that his early childhood Download trauma could happen anywhere. And from then on the sight of numbers triggered his freeze response and sent him into dissociation. With Memory Reconsolidation he gained the capacity to be calm in the presence of doing math.

I watch people tremble and shake when they trigger with their PTSD issues. Like with Susan, I often hear their stories roll out after the power has been discharged from their issues. I hurt for people who live with the terrors of PTSD. I hurt for young veterans and old veterans who have come home with an internal hell.

I know that Memory Reconsolidation works, this discovery made in a neuroscience laboratory in the year 2000. I know Memory Reconsolidation can be applied efficiently using The ICE Method I share in this book. Further, I know that ICE works even for the most highly charged peptides stored at the synapses of a person's brain. I know this about Memory Reconsolidation and The ICE Method. Now I hope to share their usefulness as broadly as possible.

I haven't had a case where Memory Reconsolidation hasn't worked. If the identify, calm and exchange steps happen with The ICE Method or with some other process, Memory Reconsolidation will happen. If the steps of Memory Reconsolidation don't occur, then a memory doesn't get reconsolidated.

When I first started sharing The ICE Method, I expected it would be easy to access agencies and organizations working with PTSD. To date, those doors have not yet opened but I feel confident they will. I look forward to when Memory Reconsolidation is known by everyone.

When I served as a pastor, I always felt a deep gratitude as I offered the blessing that closed each worship service. It comes to mind as I close this chapter on PTSD. It feels right to be calling on any traditions, all traditions, that carry words of love and compassion meant to reach the deepest corners of our life. If you or someone you know lives with PTSD – blessings for your journey. If Memory Reconsolidation and The ICE method can provide relief, I will feel such thankfulness when your PTSD turns to calm.

May the Lord bless you and keep you.
May the Lord's face shine upon you and be gracious to you.
May the Lord look upon you with favor and grant you peace.

9 – Neuroplasticity and Neurogenesis

Neuroplasticity and neurogenesis are two of the most significant discoveries in brain science. Neuroplasticity and neurogenesis have become our most popular explanation for how we can change our emotions and behaviors. But they are not the same as Memory Reconsolidation.

As both introduction and conclusion:

- Neuroplasiticy and neurogenesis *build* new brain connections.
- Memory Reconsolidation *replaces* chemistry in existing stored brain connections.

We learn when we build new brain connections. In some cases we can actually grow new brain cells during our later life – the process called neurogenesis. More commonly, the wiring grows and adapts to hook existing brain cells together in new ways. A foundational researcher in this area, Donald Hebb, coined the phrase, "neurons that fire together wire together." As we put effort into learning, and as our brain cells work on this learning process, more wiring and more synapses build to support this learning.

Imagine yourself a kid born in the United States who loves sports. You move to India and all of a sudden you have to learn cricket. All the other kids started wiring brain cells together around cricket a long time ago. For you, this game is brand new and you don't have cricket wiring. Your brain starts searching for comparisons to other experiences, and it starts wiring together new connections. You begin to create neural cricket pathways in your brain. Eventually, neuroplasticity helps you create the new habit of cricket.

Neuroplasticity is *the* way to go when you want to learn a *new* habit or skill, but neuroplasticity offers a poor approach when you want to get rid of an old habit. For old habits and old stored upset emotions, Memory Reconsolidation works in a way that neuroplasticity never can.

I really, really want you to get this paragraph. When I wrote the first sentence I stopped for a long time. If you can get this difference, you will have a profoundly more powerful and effective life. Most people don't get this distinction, so they end up stuck with adding more and more learning to their life. Learning is great, but it won't get rid of the upset emotional peptides at the base of an issue.

Whenever anyone wants to get rid of an old habit and says to me, "I know this is going to be a lot of work," I know they have a neuroplasticity mindset.

- Use neuroplasticity for new habits and learning.
- Use Memory Reconsolidation to replace old stored upset emotions that interfere with your freedom to learn

If you find yourself blocked because of old stored emotions, no new learning can remove the stored peptides. People sometimes try dozens of times to get rid of an old habit – without success. They keep using neuroplasticity to create new brain wiring, hoping they can get rid of an old habit and get on with their new life. With all their effort they create a new habit, maybe something like drinking juice instead of eating ice cream, to get them to their goal of losing weight. But building a new habit with neuroplasticity doesn't address or remove a single stored emotional peptide. Whatever emotions the person stored about living with a certain amount of weight; these emotions persist. If you don't remove those stored emotions with Memory Reconsolidation, then your new habit will always fight against your old stored emotions of fear, anger, sadness or whatever else.

Neuroplasticity does not address old stored emotional peptides.

If you have to fight stored emotions, you will need constant willpower to maintain your new neuroplastic habit.

Workarounds

When you use neuroplasticity to to overcome a problem in your life, you are creating what I call a *workaround*. A workaround is a new habit, a new set of brain wiring you create through repetitive hard work. If you want a really great book about this, I recommend *Evolve Your Brain* by Joe Dispenza[38] Dispenza writes with an easy to understand style. He has a great way of explaining what happens in your brain when you create a new habit. Neuroplasticity explains the powerful brain process that helps a kid learn to play cricket in India. But for bringing permanent calm to stored emotional upsets, neuroplasticity won't help a bit.

If you create a new habit around an old issue in your life, you don't get rid of the emotional strength of the old issue. The emotion remains and it will stay there for the rest of your life. With neuroplasticity you create a strong pathway *around* the old stored emotions so you don't get sucked into their vortex anymore. You might be successful in this endeavor, but…it's going to take constant effort. In Harry Potter, the teacher Mad Eye Moody always comes to mind when I think of this. If he says it once, he says it a thousand times, "constant vigilance, constant vigilance."

Why do you have to be constantly vigilant if you use neuroplasticity to build a workaround? Because the old stored emotional issue remains there the same as before - always ready to resurface unless you keep putting your vigilance, attention and energy into maintaining your new habit.

Once you see this distinction you'll find it obvious and life changing. But without knowing about Memory Reconsolidation, most people have no idea you can easily remove the charge on the old stored issue. Once you remove the charge, then you can actually create from freedom instead of creating as an escape from something bad.

"I get this," a friend said one night. A group of us were having dinner together, and the talk had turned to New Year Resolutions. I'd been trying to make this point about new habits and workarounds.

"I've been going to AA for fifteen years, and I've been sober for all that time. But not a day goes by I don't wish I could have a drink with you guys."

Going to AA reinforces the new neural pathway this friend decided to create fifteen years earlier. He made the choice back then because the side effect of drinking had become too costly. And by hard work and continuing to attend AA, he strengthened his wiring more and more. When he commented that he still wishes every day he could have that drink, he signaled to me that he still has stored emotions in his brain about the desire to drink. To date, he hasn't reconsolidated those stored emotional peptides. Result? Staying sober continues to take a lot of willpower.

I think much of current therapy remains consistent with what my friend experienced with Alcoholics Anonymous – building workarounds. Psychotherapist Bruce Ecker is one of the few who bases his therapy technique on the science of Memory Reconsolidation. He pretty much confirms my sense about therapy's reliance on neuroplasticity. Together with a team of other therapists they developed a new method called *Coherence Therapy*. "Before 2000, based on nearly a century of research, neuroscientists believed that the brain did not possess the capability of erasing an existing, established emotional learning from memory."[39] If Ecker is right, then therapy could do no more than help you become aware of your stored life experience. With this awareness, therapy could help you create alternative habits. Ecker calls this a "counteractive approach," based on neuroplasticity and building new brain networks. I call it building a workaround.

Many people I work with have tried traditional therapy. Most of them describe how therapy helped them gain insight and create different ways of understanding their past. The major problem, as these examples have shown, is the original stored upset emotion never reconsolidated. The upset stored emotion maintained a lock on the person no matter how many years of counseling they experienced. These emotions remained stuck until they used The ICE Method and finally reconsolidated them to a permanent state of calm.

In a recent issue of *The Neuropsychotherapist* devoted exclusively to Memory Reconsolidation, editor Matthew Dahlitz opens the journal with this question, "How often can we say therapy has been a categorical success? Welcome to our special issue on memory reconsolidation (MR)—a foundational process with the potential, if properly understood, to consistently bring about the kind of transformational change that we look for in the lives of clients."[40]

This journal volume goes on to describe five different case studies that employ Memory Reconsolidation. Each case demonstrates the removal of stored emotional upsets from the memories of their clients. The five methods differ, but each relies on the discovery of Memory Reconsolidation. Memory Reconsolidation remains a very new discovery, only at the leading edge of application in the world of health and healing. Perhaps a good way to close this chapter is to compare the development of Memory Reconsolidation with the earliest years of the automobile.

Neuroplasticity and Neurogenesis

When the Model T arrived, it changed everything about transportation. We have not yet reached this time with Memory Reconsolidation. The discovery of Memory Reconsolidation currently compares better to when the gasoline engine first entered the horse-driven world. "What do we do with this engine?"

The very first cars that arrived were creative but strange attempts to harness the engine for transportation. The Model T would come later and make internal-combustion engine cars available for the masses. We have not yet arrived at a similar point with Memory Reconsolidation. We have just reached that earliest stage where people have started to try things out, seeing what works and what doesn't work. We have an engine – Memory Reconsolidation. "How can we apply it?"

Someday, perhaps soon, someone will come up with a Model T for Memory Reconsolidation – a delivery system that puts the permanent removal of stored emotional upsets into the hands of the masses. Like with the Model T – when this happens, the world will transform.

Imagine a world where people live and operate from a place of calm. Imagine working in this environment. Imagine bringing children into this environment. Imagine schools that teach this way. Such a world will have very different priorities from our current cultural preoccupation with "pulling ourselves up by our bootstraps." Bootstraps come from a neuroplasticity worldview. Bootstraps have their place. But neuroplasticity should come second. Neuroplasticity should come *after* we reconsolidate our experiences to calm. Then we will have a free center from which to innovate and build our lives.

So, with an eye toward helping the Model T of Memory Reconsolidation come into production, I keep tinkering with The ICE Method. The more I use it, and the more I play with Memory Reconsolidation, the more I see the depth and breadth of The ICE Method. These next chapters explore some of these broader connections.

10 - Quantum

Sometime after I started using The ICE Method for myself, I began observing the open sky as a space between two points, the space with nothing in it. Not always, but often, I'd find myself drawn to a sense of infinity in that sky space. Instead of a place of nothing, this calm space in the sky would give a feeling of connection to a vast everything.

The Observer Effect

One of the foundations of quantum theory reveals that *how* we observe something influences *what* we observe. Most of us humans spend most of our lives reacting to things in our external environment, to cars, people, words, food and nature. Most of us have our attention on reacting to this physical stuff of our life. In ICE terms, our focus is on issues rather than the calm space of nothing that lies between all the points and the things of life.

In the moment I put my attention on the infinite space of the sky, the space with nothing in it, I stepped back from observing this material world. Over time, I found that when I stopped reacting to an issue, I felt that sense of calm, but also something else.

Quantum says the material world appears to us because of the way we observe it. If we don't make a conscious observation, then we don't experience a material world. (If you don't have previous experience with quantum, I've included an appendix with some starter information.) Scientists have done this experiment hundreds of times with subatomic particles called photons. When you consciously observe the photons during an experiment, they function as particles. When you don't watch them, the photons function as a wave form, light waves. This famous experiment identified what has become known as "the observer effect."

As I said, most of us never stop observing and reacting to our external world. I have helped many people become aware they can observe the space of nothing that exists *between* all the objects of our world. Most of these people say they never experienced this sensation before. I think when we observe this "nothing," we might actually be observing "everything" – at least in quantum terms.

Quantum experiments show that when we stop observing something, it returns to its wave state. Imagine standing at the beach and looking at a sand castle a child made. It's a static material thing – every time you look it looks the same. Now imagine looking at a wave coming toward the beach. Depending on the moment you observe it, you'll see something different, such as the wave first swelling, later breaking in the water and later yet crashing up on the beach. If you don't observe it, this wave carries all possibilities of the wave. When you observe it, you see one particular snapshot of the waves journey – one physical material moment in the history of the wave. Scientists call this process of observing, "collapsing the wave." The wave of all possibilities collapses down to the single one you view in a particular instant.

The ICE Method fits nicely with this quantum understanding. When an event happens in our life, we store that event based on how we participated in it, how we observed the snapshot of that event. We store our emotion with the peptides we created at the time of the event. Like the sandcastle I just described, if we keep looking back at a life event in the same way, we will keep feeling the same emotions as when the event originally took place. This is exactly what most of us do. We keep looking back the same way – and we keep feeling the same emotion. We keep creating the same material peptide chemistry because we continue observing experiences in the same way, over and over again.

ICE allows us to change our observation.

The process of ICE'ing is a process of playing with the way we observe an event. We stop looking at life the same way, over and over again. We use our conscious attention to shift our viewpoint. We actually change the chemistry stored at the synapses of a memory. We can look at this from a biochemistry perspective. We can also look from a quantum perspective.

The ICE Method from a quantum perspective:

1. When we identify an issue in ICE, we intentionally want to recreate the stored observation. This original observation goes back to the emotion we felt when the issue took place. This is like looking at the old sand castle. It appears the same every time we look.
2. Next we put our attention on the space between the physical objects, the space with nothing in it. When we do this we change our observation. Instead of continuing in our long-held reaction to an event, we step away from that observation and step into the

calm space. In quantum, this corresponds to becoming aware of the wave state of all possibilities.
3. Finally, we look back on the original issue that we identified. Now we can look from a new and different point of observation. Like the example of observing a wave at the beach, every moment we observe the wave, we observe it at a different instant in time. Depending on the observation, the wave that we see is different. For a memory, when we use ICE we stop observing from a perspective of anger, fear or sadness. We use our consciousness so now we can observe from a place of calm. This is Memory Reconsolidation from a quantum wave perspective.

In the peptide model of Memory Reconsolidation, I help people replace their upset peptides with calm ones. In this quantum understanding of Memory Reconsolidation, a person replaces their old stored observation with a new one. When I change how I observe something, the wave collapses in a different way. Something different shows up in my physical experience.

What different thing shows up when I change how I observe an old memory? In the case of Memory Reconsolidation, peptides change. Peptides change based on whether we react to the agitated peptides from the original event or the calm peptides from the space between, the space with nothing in it. When we look back at the original event, the actual physical stored emotional peptides of that event change – based solely on how we look at the event. This holds true, even when we observe the original event, years after it first happened. ICE is based on using our conscious awareness to change physical chemistry. ICE gives us a peptide based explanation – quantum give us an energy based explanation.

You can use ICE just fine without understanding a bit about quantum. So why bother with it?

More and more people who work in the area of healing, understand their work in terms of quantum energy. Paying attention to quantum creates the possibility for broader connections and broader applications for Memory Reconsolidation. I believe people who use quantum concepts in their healing can benefit by knowing the three steps of The ICE Method. Even though quantum healing methods deal directly with energy – quantum is still working with the material physical life we experience. This physical life shows up as stored emotional chemistry in the brain.

The Light Within

Recently, my wife and I attended a weekend workshop on a process called The Light Within. The developer, Kim Levinson, has a background in Reiki and other energy healing methods. As a result of a near-death experience over twenty years ago, she has dedicated her life to helping people experience and share the energy she has experienced.

"First and foremost," writes Kim in her workbook, "You must acknowledge that energy exists in all that surrounds us and all is possible. We are all connected. Give gratitude and thanks to God – the divine Source."

This is quantum shared in everyday words. In Reiki and in Kim's Light Within, practitioners feel this energy, this vibration, this light, and they share it between themselves and the people they work with.

Kim reminds people, "For those clients who are very linear thinkers and overly analytical in this type of work, please remind them not to analyze why they are having a vision or why their hands are reaching for the sky, etc. If they try to analyze it, the vision will go away."

Again, different language for what I explained earlier about ICE. If we observe (analyze) a particular situation, then our reaction focuses on that situation. If instead we can back off and let ourselves feel the energy that connects everything (become aware of a calm space) then we can have an experience of the quantum state of all possibilities. As Kim says, "You want them to let their minds go into a state of allowing."

With experience, practice and desire, we can grow to have deeper awareness of the quantum state. In Kim's words, which relate directly to quantum, "Remember, the light within has always been with us. We were born with this knowledge; we knew it in the womb. I could continue going backwards before the womb, but this is a good place to begin."

I first met Kim at a health-fair expo, and she offered me a demonstration session. I had never before experienced a practitioner having such a direct influence on my physical sensations and emotions. Even while she offered the session to me, I knew I wanted more of whatever she offered. Kim's workshop turned out to be very simple. She helped all of the dozen participants experience this source energy personally. She also gave us the ability to share it with others. I've read about quantum for many years, and attended other workshops and events along the way. I've long recognized connections between quantum and peptides and The ICE Method. The Light Within workshop gave me a greater awareness for applying this quantum field during all my ICE Method sessions.

As I keep reminding myself, my purpose in writing this book is to share the discovery of Memory Reconsolidation and offer an easy method for applying it to your life. I hope you see how quantum can expand both your awareness and your abilities for using Memory Reconsolidation in your life. Next I'd like to share one simple way to integrate quantum awareness into your ICE Method process.

Feeling an Energy Ball

I told you in Chapter Four I'd share an energetic way of becoming aware of the calm space. From Reiki to ancient Chinese Medicine to quantum energy workers in many traditions, people talk about "the energy ball." You can find plenty of places that explain the energy ball in great detail. Here's a brief introduction so you have another way to experience the calm space, the quantum field, the energy that connects us all.

Use your hands to hold an imaginary ball, something the size of a large softball, so your finger tips are a few inches apart. Allow yourself to relax (Now would be a great time to do the two points and then enter the calm state). As you relax, observe your hands and notice whatever you notice. Like Kim says about analyzing what's happening – just don't. Simply observe and be aware of what you observe. Be aware of gratitude, give thanks, notice your attention moving towards calm. See if you notice a tingling or buzzing feeling in your hands. If you do, that's fine. If you don't, that's fine.

Keep observing. Notice if you feel any sensation when you move your hands closer together and then farther apart. For some people, there's a magnetic feeling. If you notice this, fine. If you don't, that's fine too. I invite you to play with this ancient technique. I have introduced the energy ball to many people. Only a few say they've previously experienced it.

If you do notice a tingling, buzzing, magnetic pull, or heat or cold sensation you can take this as a physical awareness of the wave energy state of the quantum field. When we relax our observation from reacting to specific situations, we become aware of this field of possibilities. How can this relate to The ICE Method? Why would I include energy balls in this book?

You can always do The ICE Method by going back and forth between the upset emotion and the calm space of nothing you see between any two points. But I find that some people really like this energetic sensation in their hands, and it can serve equally well for stepping out of their upset emotion. To use an energy ball with The ICE Method try this.

1. First become aware of the energetic feeling between your hands. As time goes on, you may start noticing the energetic feeling spreading from head to toe. Let this be home base, your calm center, your quantum state awareness. You'll keep coming back to this state, with just brief excursions of observing specific stored situations that carry an upset emotion.
2. After you become aware of the energy ball, identify your upset issue as when you're doing ICE normally. Just for an example, let's say you feel anger when you identify the emotion, and you feel it in your chest. Feeling this emotion corresponds to collapsing the wave. You go from universal energy ball awareness to observing a single situation, the peptide molecule of anger and its influence on your body.
3. Then return your awareness to the energy ball. This brings your awareness away from the collapsed state (anger) and back to the quantum energy state you can feel with the energy ball – the feeling of calm – the wave state of all possibilities.
4. After you again feel the energy ball, then collapse the wave again. In other words, observe back on exactly what upset you before. When you do, you will have changed the way the wave collapses. At first, the wave collapsed according to the emotion of anger. This time when the wave collapses, the emotion feels calm, the feeling of the energy ball. The wave now collapses based on the emotion of calm, and calm peptides show up in the stored memory, replacing anger peptides. In quantum terms, the situation shows up differently because you observed it differently. In ICE Method brain chemistry terms, you just exchanged peptides.

Did we need to go to all this trouble of explaining ICE in terms of quantum? No. But when we see Memory Reconsolidation both as a chemical biological process as well as a quantum process, we get a chance to have a much bigger conversation.

During the two-day Light Within workshop I felt connections to The ICE Method popping up all throughout the weekend. Without some quantum awareness I wouldn't have conncted The ICE Method together with this experience. I have a whole chapter on Integrating ICE with existing techniques. Having some understanding of quantum deepens the connections.

In quantum techniques like The Light Within, and others I have experienced, I notice a pattern. Sometimes an intention is set for a session, and sometimes no intention is set. Then the practitioner drops into awareness of the quantum field, and by this act of changing the observation, a person's life will often change. I have noticed that quantum practitioners rarely, if ever, do a corresponding process of Memory Reconsolidation. If they did a specific process of observing back on the upset, they would be accessing the quantum field according to the requirements for Memory Reconsolidation. Along with quantum, they would be changing stored material upset peptides at synapses in the brain. I think an awareness of the steps needed to reconsolidate a memory might add to the results quantum practitioners experience. The quantum process of setting an intention and dropping into the field would remain. Understanding Memory Reconsolidation would simply provide an added awareness for use in dissolving stored emotional upsets.

If a quantum practitioner wanted to incorporate Memory Reconsolidation, it would be very simple.

1. Before moving into their awareness of the field, the practitioner would have the person specifically identify the upsetting situation, the upsetting emotion and where they feel this upset in their body.
2. After the session, the practitioner would check in and see how the person feels now about the situation, what emotion do they experience and what do they feel in their body.
3. If the person has any residual upset, the practitioner could again access the quantum field and continue the quantum process according to the identify, calm and exchange pattern of The ICE Method.

So far in this chapter we've looked at the observer effect and using quantum in a healing practice such as The Light Within. We've also looked at how to connect this quantum awareness to The ICE Method. To conclude this chapter, I want to spend a bit of time on one more insight from quantum – the Zero Point Field. It will help to explain a long-distance healing experience Anne and I had after the Light Within workshop.

A friend of Anne's and mine told us about her trouble in recovering from pneumonia. She still coughed after her illness and her stomach continued to feel upset two weeks after finishing her antibiotics. Excited after our Light Within workshop we offered to do a session with our friend – long distance – she lived a four hour drive away on the other side of Washington State.

We kept our phones on during the session, and I asked the person to report what she experienced. Anne and I used our hands and attention as we had been taught, but we were paying attention to the imaginary body of our friend, right on the table in our living room. I integrated The ICE Method by asking our friend to share emotions she felt and memories that might be arising. We would direct her attention back to the energy she was feeling and then ask her to check back on the emotions and memories again. The ICE part of the session worked very similarly to a regular ICE session. As the session progressed, our friend reported strong sensations of heat and cold, skin tingling and actual pain in her throat and spine. As she told us what she experienced, Anne and I looked at each other in amazement – her responses closely corresponded to however we paid attention to the imaginary body on our table.

I'd read before about long distance effects in quantum. Based on what scientists have discovered about quantum, it made sense to me as a possibility. This experience with our friend completed a journey for me – quantum moved from being theoretically interesting to now being experientially, completely undeniable.

Findings from the Zero Point Field

In the quantum world scientists relate matter to energy by Einstein's famous equation, $E = mc^2$. Matter and energy connect to each directly. We've used that awareness in the first part of this chapter as we paid attention to the observer effect. It turns out, though, even when you remove all available energy from a given space, it still contains more energy in that space, lots more. Again, you don't need this information to use The ICE Method, but it may increase your understanding and effectiveness.

Scientists call this fluctuating intersection between energy and the momentary flashes of particles the Zero Point Field. In this quantum field every piece of energy connects to every other piece. If something happens at one place in the Zero Point Field, the effects show up instantaneously throughout the field, holographically. Extend the results of non-locality, entanglement, and the observer effect across the universe, and you get the Zero Point Field.

A cubic meter, less than the space under your dining room table, contains enough energy to boil all the oceans of the world.[41] And because waves store information as well as transmit energy, scientists believe all the information in all the books stored in the Library of Congress could be contained in the Zero Point Field – in a space the size of a sugar cube. This information appears throughout the field, everywhere and instantaneously. Lots to absorb, but just a few perceptions about quantum can be enough to transform our perceptions forever about this material life. And it can change our perceptions of what's possible for our emotional and physical health.

In the quantum world scientists speak of vibrations instead of material things. In quantum, the explanation would use waves instead of peptides. The ICE Method makes sense either way. Peptides show up in the concrete material visible world, but they originate from non-material consciousness, information, and emotion.

Peptides form as the material result of emotions and the Zero Point Field.

Emotional peptides come from this vast universal field of inconceivable energy and incredible information.

In this view of the universe, it becomes impossible to fully separate out any single thing from the whole. One particle affects another. Change the one, and the other responds. Things get shared in the quantum world.

Light and health in the quantum world.

It has been a challenge for researchers to take findings on the subatomic level and apply them to larger objects and living organisms. One person who did just this is Fritz Albert Popp.[42] As far back as the 1970's, he had already discovered that living beings emit light waves. He measured this light in the form of tiny quantum behaving photons. He discovered that in healthy humans this light was entangled and coherent – it carried information.

The light we emit comes from interaction with the Zero Point Field.

Popp believes this provides the answer for how our bodies take shape after our conception and how we become who we are. Our biology exists in a direct relationship to the quantum field. Traditional biologists haven't been able to find a chemical or electrical answer for how the body can coordinate 50-100 trillion cells, each undergoing something like 100,000 chemical reactions per second. The standard explanation of electrical conduction through brain cells and nerve cells happens far too slowly to explain something like a baseball batter hitting a fastball pitch. Quantum entanglement offers an explanation for this amazing coordination between our minds and the cells of our bodies.

In further tests, Popp explored the relationship between a person's health and the characteristics of the light they emit. He compared the light emitted by healthy people to people with cancer and people with multiple sclerosis. Compared to healthy people, cancer sufferers emitted less light. For those suffering from cancer, they had too little light (too little information) in their bodies to coordinate healthy cellular activity. One can imagine that without proper coordination, cells could begin to grow haphazardly without the necessary healthy template of information being provided by the light waves. Many researchers believe this haphazard growth is exactly what happens in the development of cancer cells.

How could this information about light help a person use The ICE Method? All along we've said that paying attention to stored emotional upsets and replacing them with calm allows the body to operate in a state of rest and restoration. Memory Reconsolidation replaces energy-draining upsets with healing calm. Popp might say it helps a person get their light right.

In multiple sclerosis it turns out that people take in and emit more light (more information) than healthy people. When people take in too much light it corresponds to taking in too much organization and control. This light is also less coherent, less patterned, more disturbed. As the body accepts too much confused information from its external environment it restricts the body's systems with too many instructions. In this restrictive environment, the body cannot freely maintain health. Interestingly, multiple sclerosis is one of the diseases on the long list of autoimmune disorders.

In autoimmunity, internal stress and a stuck fight/flight/freeze response have turned the body's immune system against itself.[43] Popp's studies of stress confirmed that a person's light emissions rise when they experience stress. In chronic autoimmunity terms, the body has lost its ability to distinguish between external and internal threats; the body has lost its freedom to react appropriately to the environment. In terms of quantum light, the body absorbs too much light, too much

Quantum

information, too many conditions and too many constraints. It would make sense that one of the autoimmune characteristics is inflammation, the body's reaction to bombardment by the external environment – by the quantum field. Entering the calm state and reconsolidating stored upsets, once again, helps a person get their light right.

Not long ago I helped a woman reconsolidate her early-childhood PTSD memories. A few days later she called to tell me how she was doing,

"And my allergies are better, too," she added after telling me that some normally stressful events in her family no longer triggered her anxiety.

This woman works as a health care provider in Oklahoma, so she could easily talk about her allergies in terms of her immune system.

"It makes sense if my immune system was protecting me from all the grief I've stored in my life, it wouldn't be as strong for helping me out with allergies. I was surprised how getting calm about my childhood made an immediate difference in my physical health."

We could talk about peptides, quantum waves or photon light. Whatever explanation we prefer, something has become right and calm for this woman in her life. As a result, her physical health has improved.

Explain it any way you want; as long as you do the three steps of Memory Reconsolidation, you are transforming light, peptides, energy, matter and possibly more. Ultimately, whatever explanation we use, this woman can breathe easier about both her memories and her allergies.

Quantum changes our scientific worldview from isolation and separation to entanglement and infinite cooperation. In the quantum world we humans, just like subatomic particles, exist as pure energy and pure information. We connect to past and future as much as to this present moment. What we observe in this material moment of our existence happens because of our consciousness, because of the way we observe.

If we allow ourselves to embrace this quantum understanding, we can envision our material lives unfolding as a direct result of our consciousness. The ICE Method is consistent with this quantum understanding – body follows mind. Consciousness creates our experience in this material world. Isolation, separateness, individuality are all illusion. Pay attention to your mind and your energy. Your body follows your mind.

As I said at the start of this discussion, quantum is entirely optional for your success in using The ICE Method. Quantum does explain, though, why our conscious attention can have such an enormous impact on how we experience our emotional and physical reality.

We *are* our consciousness – in quantum words, what we get is what we see.

If you have any familiarity with science, you know that for the past 300 years we lived with a huge split between science and religion. With the understanding of quantum, this split has begun to heal. If we wish, we now can choose to understand that both science and religion depend on the way we observe. Old science and old religion were both like particles – waves that had collapsed to a single possibility. Stuck emotions of anger and fear made these possibilities seem mutually exclusive. As both a pastor and an engineer, I have lived on both sides of this old fence.

Now with quantum we understand that everything we observe shows up because of the way we observe. For more and more people, religion and science increasingly share common ground. In this next chapter we take a brief look at the spirit side of peptides.

11 – A Spirit Side of Peptides

Some people I work with ask if The ICE Method is a spiritual practice.

"Not directly," I answer, "but ICE can be a tool for whatever path you follow. ICE removes stuck stuff – stuck peptides, and that can make the spiritual path feel more open."

That reminder to self again:

I can share the scientific finding of Memory Reconsolidation and show a simple technique for permanently exchanging upset emotional peptides with calm ones.

So why a chapter on spirituality? Because for a significant number of people, the spiritual connections begin naturally arising as The ICE Method and calm become a way of life.

As I've already said, once I became aware of The ICE Method, I felt instantly enchanted. And that enchantment has only grown deeper and stronger for me as ICE continues integrating into the core of who I am.

As I looked between the two points to the space that has nothing in it, I found this feeling more and more like a meditational practice. Once I reconsolidated a charged issue, I'd often find myself observing the sky in the distance, extending that calm space toward the distant heavens and observing whatever showed up; emotions, physical sensations, memories or insights.

After a certain amount of experience with ICE, I became aware of connections to the quantum physics worldview I described in the last chapter. As I continued to observe that space with "nothing" in it, I started sensing an awareness, perhaps of this energy that scientists call the Zero Point Field. As charged peptides dropped out of my life, this calm space began feeling richer and richer. The calm space grew beyond just a place to pick up emotionally uncharged peptides. A deeper sense of both science and spirit began to arise.

Non-Attachment

As my experience accumulated I realized something else. Whenever we ICE an issue to calm, we become emotionally "unattached" to that experience. Perhaps we can suddenly speak calmly in public, because no terror remains in the experience. Or we can forgive a family member for a long-held upset, because the anger has gone from the memory. Maybe we can relate better to a divorced partner because we have no fear left in the events of the past.

"Non-attachment" arises naturally when we replace agitated peptides with calm peptides. Many spiritual practices have non-attachment as their goal. The non-attachment goal makes good sense to me. How can you feel at peace if you feel "attached," or emotionally reactive to something or someone? If you react to something or someone in your life, then you end up dependent on how that person feels. If you live in reaction to another, you can only feel peaceful if they feel peaceful. Just look as far as a family member or friend. If one person feels highly agitated, most of the other people will feel agitated in response. Being around anxiety does not usually promote a sense of peace - but it can if you ICE. When you reconsolidate whatever shows up as anxious, you can actually live from a peaceful state. You can have this peace even when you find yourself in the presence of anxiety or other upset. As long as you have no immediate present physical danger, you can have this calm. By now you know where I'm headed. ICE your life. When you do, you become non-attached to whatever you used to find yourself reacting to in the past.

Spirituality places great emphasis on non-attachment. The great ones had this – Jesus – Buddha – Gandhi – Theresa - Tutu – King. I have more of this non-attachment than I did before – but I don't have it completely. Just a moment ago I clicked over to the Internet to find a resource and check out a thought for this chapter. My email page popped up first.

I see an announcement for a class a colleague is offering, and I click the email open. A week ago this friend and I had been on the phone, and I'd helped him ICE through an issue. I was also testing out a new technique for accessing calm.

A Spirit Side of Peptides

There in his announcement I read the words and spirit of what I'd shared with him, right at the top. Bam – immediately I lose my calm. When you play the calm game long enough, the feeling of non-calm hits you right away: very noticeable.

I stop reading and start identifying. "He's taking my material."

I'm "mature" enough to recognize the immaturity of this thought. And I completely realize that this new thing I shared with my friend came from something shared with me only a few days earlier by another person.

But the feeling is there.

Instead of denying the feeling, I grab it and start squeezing it for whatever I can identify. Before I learned ICE I would have run from these feelings, denying them as quickly as possible so I could move on. Now, with ICE, I almost always run toward my upsets, knowing there's something new to bring to calm.

My old issue with "control" shows up again. Surprise, surprise. I've reconsolidated plenty of peptides around my life experiences with control, and I know those which became calm in the past remain calm to this day. But now some new synapses just activated. I realize a feeling that I want to control The ICE Method: I want everything to funnel out through me. I want it to go through me first, and then out to the broader world. Wow. Not a mature feeling, but a big realization.

Next, almost immediately, I realize what an insufficient being I would be for having everything go through me first and then out to the rest of the world. I don't have enough organization, enough smarts, enough diversity. I recognize past opportunities that could have been so much more useful to people if someone did what my colleague just did – take the insight and run with it.

Next I recognize I am not the source of ICE and I am not the source of what I continue to become aware of. I have one voice within the source, but I am not the source. My old control issue, the emotion of fear, is not helping me here. These old stored peptides get in the way of me celebrating my colleague and supporting his amazing work to help grow great lives. Do I feel open to reconsolidating these peptides to calm? Yes!

Having identified, I use the two points and head back out to the calm space. I notice the deepening feeling go through my chest as it always does when I return to the calm state. I observe this space in the sky that opens me to this awareness of non-reactivity. Body chemistry changes to calm. Mind reverts back to calm.

Finally I observe back on this email that just triggered me, and I observe all that I identified, and I exchange peptides. And it all goes to calm. I read my colleagues words again. I feel more deeply aware that what I received and shared with this person is not my possession at all. It came as gift, and whatever I received can pass forward as gift. The person who shared her method with me already has this maturity. She knows that what she has to offer came first as a gift to her. Her peptides about sharing hold no charge other than excitement. And now mine feel that way too.

A little embarrassing to write this? Yes, of course. But I want you to see that the first rising of an issue often sparks a reactivity in us. I felt surprise when I first read the email. Then when I paid attention I felt the emotion of fear that The ICE Method would spin out of my control. As soon as I reflected on this, I realized the "immaturity" of the feeling, the "embarrassment" – and the tendency to deny and run away from it.

When you run away emotionally, activated peptides won't reconsolidate. They will reglue the same way and they will wait in your synapses until they trigger you again. If you don't ICE your upsets or reconsolidate them in some other way, they'll glue back down in the same pattern. They will wait for the rest of your life, ready to spark your upset the next time they get activated. According to scientific understanding your brain really does work this way. Most people struggle to figure out ways around their issue, like running away or building new habits. If you want simplicity and effectiveness, you can use Memory Reconsolidation to permanently replace the upsets.

How do I feel now after ICE'ing this upset I just became aware of? I feel non-attached to my colleague sending out his email. Non-attachment does not feel the same to me as spirituality. Non-attachment opens space, though, and this space can potentially fill with a sense of spirit.

What do I feel in place of the fear that arose a few moments ago? I feel peaceful. I feel gratitude for this man's lifelong endeavor to probe consciousness for himself, to share his journey with others and for his burning desire to help individuals raise their consciousness. I feel inspired and in awe of his passion and creativity. I like these non-attached feelings so much better than the fear feeling that triggered just a few moments ago.

The ICE Method provides a dependable mechanical path for growing non-attachment in your life.

In spiritual terms what I feel for my colleague and friend is closer to compassion and love. At the base of most spiritual and religious expressions, compassion and love typically serve as the foundation. Those who come to deeply know compassion call it easy and natural. I think they speak from the hindsight of a long journey. ICE can speed this journey. ICE can help you more quickly develop calm, non-attachment, and compassion.

Birthright Calm

At some point in a session I often start explaining we have a birthright state which is calm. It's a spirit statement, and also a quantum statement. A lot of people find it resonates. Perhaps you'll find it useful too.

Before our conception, we had no peptides to react to. We all have this birthright place of calm from before our conception – a place and time before reactive peptides became a part of our life. Spiritual traditions talk about this in terms of the universe and love and consciousness. Now some quantum scientists use the same language, that our universe organizes around love; that consciousness came before the development of physical matter.[44,45] When I talk about birthright calm, some people recognize these intersections with spirit. Others don't have spirit as part of their language. But everyone gets this picture of how our emotional peptides don't begin accumulating until our brain starts developing.

Emotional peptides then start storing as soon as we begin our journey in the womb. We store reactions to our environment beginning before our birth. In fact, the fastest time of our brain development in our entire life happens during our time in the womb. We store a lot during the first nine months of our existence.

"When we draw our last breath," I tell people, "we will return to this birthright of calm. We will experience no more reactive peptides. In between our conception and our death, we live in a world of reactive peptides.

"When you use The ICE Method," I continue, "you regain your birthright calm right here in the middle of your life experience. The more you ICE away old stored peptides, the more of your birthright calm you get to enjoy again, right now in your daily life."

At this point, we usually do a little exercise to create a calm house image, or a calm garden, a calm beach or whatever image works as a visualized place of this birthright calm. "If you wish, you can live from this place from now on," I tell them, "with exceptions.

"When the exceptions arise, when you react to stored peptides, imagine this happening *outside* of your calm place. Go *outside* of your calm place and ICE this new upset back to calm. Once you do then notice you can bring that reactive thing inside your calm place. Once it feels truly calm, it no longer causes a reaction, and it can exist inside and alongside your birthright calm."

In spiritual terms, this process often goes by the name of "non-attachment." Conceivably, if a person becomes non-attached to all their stored reactivities, they might end up with more openness to the spiritual experience of complete oneness with the universe. Some call this enlightenment. ICE won't enlighten you, but it can help open the space of non-attachment. And that space might make enlightenment more likely. The ICE Method provides a tool for those on a spiritual journey, a simple, mechanical and powerful process for becoming non-reactive to stored peptides.

Our six-year dream

I'll get back to Memory Reconsolidation, but for a moment I want to pay more attention to this birthright calm. Our birthright calm starts getting other inputs once the peptides start storing in the womb. For the first six-or-so years of our life, as I mentioned in Chapter Seven, we absorb these emotional peptides while in a hypnotic brain state. This theta-brain-wave state beats at a slow four to seven cycles per second. In this state you absorb experiences without the kind of reflection that starts happening after about the age of six.

This collection of emotions gets stored in the synapses between our brain cells. The peptides stored during these first six years form the framework for what we judge as safe, and what we perceive as dangerous. These become our automatic settings for our comfort range. We can act outside this comfort range or act against what's comfortable, but when we do, it will take effort, and we'll be activating our fight/flight/freeze danger peptides. Think for a few moments and if you're human, I think you'll find examples of this in your life.

If we start using The ICE Method, we get a simple way for picturing how this part of life works – peptides. When I started using The ICE Method for myself, I was stunned a few weeks later when I realized how completely my life had been lived in reaction to stored peptides. I felt such amazement and gratitude for this awareness of Memory Reconsolidation. Finally something could actually reveal and address this "operating program" I had stored for my whole life. When I started using ICE with other people, I found that every one of them had also lived out of reactions to stored reactive emotional peptides. Some of us have Downloads that allow us to function successfully. Others have Downloads that propel us towards undesired results. Either way though, successful or not, we live in reaction to the stored peptides that created our safe and danger settings long ago in our early childhood.

This "peptide operating system" came as a new realization for me. My worldview before Memory Reconsolidation seemed like that of most people I experience – we need to work hard to create the lives we want. This now seems partially true to me. The hidden part, the part that's really hard to see without Memory Reconsolidation, is that almost everything we build, we do as a reaction to our earliest storage about safe and dangerous. The positive and the negative, we do them both to satisfy the stored peptides from early life that created our safe and danger zones.

Few of us live from a true state of freedom.
Most of us live from a state of reactivity to old stored peptides.

I make no judgment in this observation. It just seems true for me and for almost everyone I meet. How do we gain back our freedom?

If we want a free life,
we need to reconsolidate stored peptides.

If we want freedom, we must recover our birthright sense of calm. In whatever ways we do not experience this birthright calm we live *attached* to something other than this calm. Non-attachment gets discussed a lot in spirituality and in religious traditions. The ICE

Method provides a simple and direct method of experiencing non-attachment. We can live non-attached to specific experiences of our life that used to carry emotional charge. And we can become non-attached from the Download of our early years. These all exist as stored peptides that can reconsolidate to calm.

A new theta dream?

Somewhere around the age of six, our waking brain wave frequency speeds up. When it speeds up we gain the power of reflection. Even though we gain the power of reflection and analysis, most of us still spend the rest of our lives reacting to what we loaded and stored during our first six years. This is why The ICE Method can be so helpful. We can free ourselves from reacting to old stored peptides, even the early peptides from our first six years.

If we actually ICE everything to calm, if we become "non-attached," then what?

The short answer is, we're free. Free to live non-reactively. Free to create.

The longer answer is we often don't know how to live with this new freedom. We have lived for so long in reaction to stored emotional upsets that we feel clueless about what to do or what to be when we finally experience non-attachment and freedom.

I used to feel I'd shared all I could about The ICE Method when a person gained the tools to non-attach from whatever showed up in their life. The ICE Method does that one little thing I've kept coming back to this whole book – it uses Memory Reconsolidation to replace stored upset emotional peptides with calm ones.

As time went on I became aware we can re-enter this childhood theta state at will. This is not new information, just new to me.

What if we could re-enter that early-years' theta state again as adults after we ICE ourselves to calm? We can, and there are many techniques to do so. Hypnotists can induce theta state. People skilled at meditation and yoga can enter theta state. And processes exist that entrain the brain to follow a frequency and settle into theta state. Indigenous cultures from around the world have used the sound of drums and rattles beating at four beats per second to entice the brain-wave state into theta frequency. This is the state of trance and journeys

A Spirit Side of Peptides

in native traditions. These traditional practices go back at least tens of thousands of years.[46]

The various traditional practices around the world have many similarities. If you want to use this theta wave state for building a path forward, most of the techniques advocate having a question to explore or an intention to pursue as you enter into the trance state. We all have our beliefs about how the world works, but from modern physics to ancient spirituality, these ways of looking at the world suggest we can receive direct revelation beyond the material realm of our everyday living.[47,48]

None of the resources I've found about the theta-wave state make any mention of Memory Reconsolidation. What a difference Memory Reconsolidation could make. The knowledge of how Memory Reconsolidation works adds something new to this process of dream building, path-finding or whatever you want to call it.

It does not matter whether we believe this material realm holds everything that exists or whether we feel we've experienced an enlightened connection with spiritual oneness – if we carry stored emotional upsets in our life, we will live in reaction to the upsets. Think of sages and gurus who end up in trouble because of their idiosyncratic behaviors. The same can happen for Christian pastors and Catholic priests. In the indigenous traditions, the same risks existed for those on spiritual paths. Sandra Ingerman and Hank Wesserman describe five classes of shamans.[49] Look at these examples from a peptide perspective, and you'll see that stored peptides even shape the characteristics of a shaman. Direct revelation for shamans? Yes. Spiritual enlightenment? Yes. Reactivity to stored peptides? Also yes.

**If a person continues to live in reactivity
to stored emotional peptides,
their life will reflect this condition.**

The first classification of shamans is the *dangerous* type. They do terrible deeds, "because in an infantile way they are truly fearful of the environment and strike out against it."[50] The second class of shaman operates according to *strict tradition*. "They may be effective in some ways but unable to cope with anything they have not seen before or have not been taught to do." You see the fear in these two first classes of shamans. Yes, they have the experience of direct revelation, but they still live in reaction to stored upset emotional peptides. The authors continue through the classes until they reach the fifth class, the "philosophically-oriented" shaman. "They are self-realized masters of their trade. They do not necessarily follow the rules because they know how to do things their own way and do not rely on the traditions to bolster them."[51]

Ingerman and Wesserman conclude their description with these helpful words: "These differences do not apply only to shamans but to people in many walks of life: business people, helping professionals, homemakers, and modern visionaries."[52] In other words, as we've already noted – peptides matter to all of us, no matter how *spiritual* or how *worldly* our perspective on life. (In Chapter 13 I'll share a few of the specific methods traditional people use to neutralize charged memories.)

Understanding we can access a theta-wave state later in life may give us a conscious opportunity to *redream* our lives. If we reconsolidate and reach a greater state of non-attachment, then we can enter this new dream and create from a place of freedom.

My experience from working with The ICE Method is that most of us get our early peptide Download and then continue living from this Download for the rest of our lives. I feel I lived that way until a few years ago when I became aware of Memory Reconsolidation and started ICE'ing my life. And I still find that slivers of my Download show up from time to time. As they arise, I ICE. What I can say for myself is that I now have a lot less Download peptides that I react to.

For some people, for whatever reason, a time in life arises when people begin to question their Download and seek alternatives. If they don't come upon Memory Reconsolidation in some form, this questioning can be a hard time, a struggle to build new neural pathways to overcome the old stored Download. If they do come upon Memory Reconsolidation, they can find non-attachment and freedom. If a person has the good fortune to come to calm, then spending time in theta-wave state may be a useful way to create new and free possibilities for living.

Maybe I've written enough on this topic. If this helps, fantastic; if not, just remember the purpose of this book - introducing Memory Reconsolidation, peptides, and the simple method of ICE for bringing this scientific discovery into your life. Use what you find useful to your own journey of life.

12 – Death

This chapter can be short. Do you feel comfortable with your coming death? If not, let's talk: About this imminent thing – our death, which was certain since our birth. If you live as most of us do, we keep death far from present consciousness.

You could ICE everything which does not feel calm about your dying. When you do, you will have gained an enormous freedom to live. Many of the spiritual traditions speak of this life freedom that comes in the wake of this death freedom.

What might you ICE? Whatever comes up. Take it as it comes. Start with your own primary emotion about death. Do you feel anger, fear, sadness or something else? Where do you feel this in your body? What memories arise – about Aunt Mary, a friend with a terminal illness, a gruesome accident you saw, a movie scene? Take them one by one. Emotions. Locations. Memories. Anticipations. Continue until you feel calm about dying.

Then start testing out your new found calm about your dying. ICE whatever comes up that does not feel calm in your imagination. At some point you'll have a true freedom around your death. You will feel "non-attached" to this inevitable event. You will have a far greater capacity to live freely in the present moment rather than fearfully about your future death.

Exceptions will almost certainly arise from time to time. ICE these as they show up in your life. In due course you will gain an enormous freedom in living, now that you no longer fear your dying.

I feel grateful I did this exercise for my own life. I repeat it as needed.

Ed and I had completed two ICE sessions when he emailed to set up a third. Our earlier Skype meetings had helped him get over what he called "melancholy," a low-grade long term depression that had dogged him since college. Ed had contacted me from his home in Northern Maine from the middle of one of the darkest coldest winters on record. I wondered if his depression had returned.

Soon after our call begins, Ed tells me he wants to start doing more volunteering. "I'm spending too much time wondering if this is 'all there is.' I don't feel the melancholy anymore, but I want something to fill my time."

I hear the words "fill my time," and make a little checkmark in my mind as I continue to listen.

"Ed," I say when he has explained his situation, "working at the homeless shelter in your town would be great. But maybe it would be good if you first use The ICE Method on your feelings about death."

On the screen I see Ed's face change to a huge look of surprise.

"The traditions talk a lot about getting calm about death. If you ICE your death you'll be free to make any choice you want. You can make choices not based on just 'filling your time.'"

So begins a wonderful session. We do very little actual ICE'ing during the session – Ed has already done a lot of this work himself. Instead we share thoughts and ideas about living from calm, living with non-attachment and living without anger, fear or sadness about death. We're talking about ICE as a tool for Ed to live the life he desires.

"If you do ICE your peptides about death," I say to Ed, "I think you'll get to live out of freedom and compassion. It's a very different thing to do your volunteering from compassion instead of filling time to avoid depression."

I tell Ed about my own experience of reacting to peptides. I grew up with Download peptides that made me focus on social justice. I did many good social projects but underneath all my action was the emotion of anger. Once I paid attention to my death and ICE'd my upsets, I gained a deeper peace in my life. I still do social action, but not from anger anymore.

I share a story with Ed. "A long time ago I heard a story about Mother Teresa. I never understood it until after I ICE'd my death. Mother Teresa was once asked if she would participate in an anti-war protest. She refused. When asked why, she replied, 'I will not participate in an anti-war protest, but I will participate in a Peace March.'"

"Ed, those are the calm peptides speaking, not the angry ones."

After a moment I ask Ed. "Do you want to start ICE'ing your death?"

"I didn't think I'd be ICE'ing my death today! But, yes, I want to do it."

Ed says he feels fear, but also sadness, and also a feeling of anger as well. The sadness and fear he notices in his stomach. The anger he feels in shoulders. He spends a few moments exploring memories and experiences about death and dying. We do a couple of rounds of ICE, and he feels noticeably calmer.

"If you want to be completely free about living," I tell Ed, "keep checking for whatever doesn't feel calm about death and dying. Keep ICE'ing whatever shows up – you'll transform your life."

Ed's been using ICE for a lot of things in his life. Our conversation today has taken a deeper turn.

"So, Ed," I ask. "This calm you feel right now. Is this what you want for your life?"

"It is," he replies. "I'm starting to see how ICE can be for how I live instead of just for how I solve problems."

"That's wonderful. I want to suggest a game." I tell him. "If you end up in a situation where you can't get back to calm by yourself, you call me and I'll help you find your calm again. Explore everything and anything that's not calm in your life – and reconsolidate whatever shows up. If you start playing that game right now you'll have a life of calm from this moment forward. If you get stuck – just let me know and I'll help you get back to ICE'ing again."

"I'd feel bad about calling you all the time."

"Not after ten. And not before eight! Any other time just let me know when you get stuck. If you keep ICE'ing to calm, you'll find yourself feeling reactive less and less often, even when you focus on your death."

"Okay, I'll do it. If I get stuck I'll call."

13 – Integrating ICE with Existing Methods

A wicker chair enfolds me. My feet rest on hardwood here at Inner Mountain Healing Arts in Chelan. Many practitioners have worked here over the years, and hundreds of people have benefitted from the practitioners of this place. I have enjoyed the invitation to share The ICE Method from Inner Mountain the past two years. Now I want to sit here while I write this chapter, thankful and aware of the tradition of healing throughout the world we live in; back through ages upon ages. I want to sit here in the humble awareness of mind, body and spirit and the loving attention that has been given towards wellness, probably for as long as we humans have had consciousness.

As I wrote in Chapter Nine, Memory Reconsolidation has not yet reached a comparable stage to the Model T. We don't yet have a widespread new modality that has captured everyone's attention. Remembering why I wrote this book, I want to turn now to some thoughts on how an awareness of Memory Reconsolidation might integrate with the healing work that people already do. That very specific contribution, again, that I feel I have to offer: I can share the discovery of Memory Reconsolidation and the knowledge of how peptides instruct both body and mind. And I can offer the simple ICE Method as a way for people to bring permanent calm to their stored upsets. Here are some thoughts for using Memory Reconsolidation in different applications.

Massage

A friend of ours from when we lived in Michigan has been doing massage for years. After we exchanged some ICE Method sessions I ask her thoughts on possible intersections between her work and The ICE Method.

"The best sessions," Kerry reflects, "often happen when people really share what's going on in their life before we start the massage."

"I'm sure your massages bring calm to everyone you work with," I reply. "Maybe the reason massages feel extra special when people share is they identified and activated synapses in their brain and body."

I ask Kerry, "What do you think would happen if you specifically checked in with a person on what they had shared with you before the massage? What if you asked them to go back and check on exactly what they had identified – whatever emotions, experiences, or bodily sensations they'd shared with you before their massage? If they did that within the four-hour activation window, they would permanently reconsolidate whatever peptides they had activated. Massage would be the calm state, and they would Identify before the calming massage, and then Exchange after the massage."

Craniosacral Therapy

At a workshop both of us are attending, I sit down to lunch with a craniosacral therapist.

As we share our experiences he tells me, "Craniosacral has a technique that sounds like it might already be doing Memory Reconsolidation. Sometimes during a session I have a conversation with people and ask them what they're experiencing during the session. As I work, I keep checking in with them."

"Yes, that sounds like the Identify, Calm, and Exchange steps."

Here's a situation where synapses that hold memory get activated during a calming practice of craniosacral therapy. When a therapist asks the person to keep checking back on what they notice, it will cause stored peptides to replace at synapses in the brain and at nerve connections in the body.

Knowing the science of Memory Reconsolidation gives a picture of what happens in the brain when we feel upset emotions. Adding this knowledge might increase the ease and effectiveness for craniosacral therapy to deal with agitated memories. From our lunchtime talk, it sounds like nothing would need to change in the way this therapist does his sessions. He now has the additional awareness of Memory Reconsolidation. The knowledge can complement what he already does.

Journaling

Since ancient times, writing has provided untold numbers with solace and healing. Sometimes people write free form in their journals.

Other times people follow specific instructions. Research psychologist James Pennebaker found that people who journaled for 20 minutes a day about the deepest emotions of their issues would often heal if they did this for four days straight. Immune system function would often improve.[53]

What if we knew that the process of permanently calming our upsets comes from the brain process of Memory Reconsolidation? Writing which identifies the upset, brings us to calm, and then revisits the upset within four hours will bring calm to a person's life.

We can journal to record our history. We can journal for insight. We can journal as a discipline. If we want to journal for emotional healing, if we want to bring calm to stored emotional upsets, then the journaling that provides the most benefit will consciously include a process of identifying, calming, and exchanging peptides.

If we know Memory Reconsolidation, we can take the mystery out of journaling for emotional healing. Compared to a person who doesn't know these three steps, a person who knows Memory Reconsolidation will experience more calming of their life when they journal.

Qi Gong

John Neff[54] from Leavenworth Washington is a person I could spend hours and days talking with. Besides being a passionate promoter of Qi-Gong, he studied for a doctorate in divinity in Berkeley, California, the same place where I studied to become a pastor. And he's fascinated by the science of body and mind. My wife and I signed up for an eight-week Qi-Gong class John offered last year, gaining an introduction to this ancient healing practice.

After John read my first book, *Fibromyalgia Relief* he called me to get together for tea. "In QiGong we're exchanging peptides too!"

"I haven't heard of Memory Reconsolidation before," he tells me, "but it clearly takes place in Qi-Gong."

"We have a practice of scanning the body and paying careful attention to every body part. In paying attention to the body, you become aware of emotions. Memories and experiences can come to mind."

John then describes the next part of this exercise. It matches and completes the steps required for memories to reconsolidate. "After you scan, you 'sink' your energy downward through the feet and then return to an area of tension or contraction to 'dissolve' it. Dissolving happens by simply placing your deeply relaxed intention and attention on this area of stress."

Qi-Gong has developed over thousands of years. Under the patiently observing eyes of masters, an enormous body of practice and knowledge accumulated. And scientific studies reveal more and more Western verifications of what practitioners have long known – Qi-Gong provides powerful benefits for bodily health, physical longevity and the well-being of our heart, mind and spirit.

What's the value of Memory Reconsolidation to Qi-Gong? When we know what happens at the synapses of the brain to bring about permanent emotional relief, we gain a more focused picture of what happens when we do Qi-Gong.

The intricate practice of Qi-Gong has way more going on than just Memory Reconsolidation. But knowing the part where Memory Reconsolidation happens can help people have a more powerful experience whenever they deal with issues of stored emotional upsets.

Acupuncture

Catherine Freeman[55] and I finish another session together and she tells me again how much she enjoys me offering The ICE Method while she does acupuncture with her patients.

When I ICE with someone, I always ask where a person feels sensations in their body. In my ICE Method mind, I think about peptides. In Catherine's acupuncture mind, each location holds layers of meaning. As bodily sensations activate for people during ICE, Catherine does acupuncture and helps people experience more profound calm, even making energetic connections that deepen their personal work. As we go back and forth between identifying upsets and exchanging peptides, acupuncture works right alongside of The ICE Method process.

I've done a number of sessions together with Catherine. Our connection has been a mutual appreciation for the science of how the brain and body work. Her language follows the traditions of energy meridians and Chinese medicine. The Western science language of how the brain reconsolidates memories makes consistent sense with her own training and experience. Memory Reconsolidation provides a Western story for how the brain works, based on peptides. Yet everything is energy as well as matter. Catherine sees the connections, and the people she serves receive the benefit.

Christian Worship

Sojourners restaurant in Chelan. Back booth. Pepperoni pizza. I walk two blocks from my house to get here. Pastor Paul Palumbo[56] walks two blocks from the other direction. Some of my favorite conversations in our little town happen right here. Although I'm no longer a pastor, if I were, I'd wish to be like Paul. He seems equally comfortable organizing a food bank, sitting in a bar with a troubled community member, or leading the worship service on Sunday morning. Today we find ourselves talking about worship.

"We have some folks in the congregation who have really immersed themselves in the worship service. When they find themselves in a difficult situation during the week they start reminding themselves of the Kyrie."

The Kyrie is a part of the worship service that repeats the words of scripture, "Lord, have mercy."

"And when they start repeating the Kyrie, they feel less stressed. And then when they come back to church and share what they experienced, they find they haven't stored that stress."

Paul and I have talked about Memory Reconsolidation many times together. "Sounds like saying the Kyrie is the calm space."

"Or the calm space is where you experience the Lord having mercy!" Paul turns my phrase around.

"I think this is a little different from Memory Reconsolidation," I say, "because it's bringing calm at the instant of the issue. There's no stored memory to activate. But it seems like the Kyrie, or the calm state, is keeping that issue from ever storing as an upset.

"When a memory originally stores," I continue, "brain researchers call that *consolidating* the memory. Memory Reconsolidation discovered that you could activate an old memory and then it would have to reconsolidate to stay a memory. So maybe saying the Kyrie is enough to change the original emotion of how that experience gets stored."

I ask Paul to think with me about another part of the Sunday service. In the Lutheran Church and in many others churches the service often begins with *Confession and Forgiveness*.

"Paul, I think you could do Memory Reconsolidation every Sunday. If you took just a moment for people to identify their issues before they said the Confession; that would activate synapses. And the words of the confession talk about the mercy of Almighty God. That's the calm space again.

"All they'd need," I finish, "is to exchange peptides after saying the confession. If you said something like, 'Now look back at the issues you brought to God this week. Look back and see how the Spirit of the Lord is working on these issues.'"

Paul is listening and thinking.

"That would be ICE," I tell him, "in a different language, the language of worship. Instead of Confession and Forgiveness being a general statement, it could also be very specific, and it could help people get a permanent sense of calm about whatever troubled them during the previous week."

I don't know if Paul or any other pastor will ever build their worship service around Memory Reconsolidation. I know for myself that in the years I served as a pastor, I never had Memory Reconsolidation in my mind. If I did, though, I know I could have been far more effective in the counseling and caring work I did in the congregations I served.

If a pastor were interested in using Memory Reconsolidation, no explanation would be needed for the congregation. Just staying attentive to helping a person identify upsets in their life would be a natural activity for most pastors. That identification activates peptides at the synaptic level. Offering a prayer that brings a person to calm would also be a natural activity for a pastor. The difference comes in getting a person to observe back on exactly what they found upsetting. When these three steps happen within a four-hour window of time, memories will reconsolidate and peace will replace upsets. Whether you call it Memory Reconsolidation or the Peace of God it seems like both good science and holy work.

Psychotheraphy and Coherence Therapy

The first book ever on the clinical application of Memory Reconsolidation was published only in 2012 by Bruce Ecker, Robin Ticic, and Laurel Hulley.[57] Before Ecker and Hulley learned of Memory Reconsolidation they had already developed Coherence Therapy, a new system that grew out of observing techniques that were producing lasting change for clients. When they learned of Memory Reconsolidation, they found a neurobiological explanation for what they had pieced together from practice and observation.

The first two sentences of *Unlocking The Emotional Brain* tell what a decisive improvement Memory Reconsolidation offers.

> What we therapists find most fulfilling are those pivotal sessions in which a client experiences a deeply felt shift that dispels longstanding negative emotional patterns and symptoms. Bringing about such decisive, liberating results for our clients sustains us, but the alchemy that produces these life-changing shifts has been something of a mystery, allowing them to come about only unpredictably in the course of many months or years of sessions."[58]

Memory Reconsolidation solves the mystery of how longstanding negative emotional patterns and symptoms get relieved. Identify. Calm. Exchange. For therapists, Memory Reconsolidation provides the answer to why therapy works when it works. Memory Reconsolidation also explains the times when therapy doesn't work – when stuck peptides did not exchange with calm.

Coherence Therapy developed as a tool for trained psychotherapists. The descriptive language differs from ICE, but that confirms the point of this whole chapter: integrating Memory Reconsolidation into existing practices. Emotional upsets calm when the steps of Memory Reconsolidation happen no matter what language we use. Thanks to Bruce Ecker and the Coherence Therapy team for their groundbreaking work in bringing Memory Reconsolidation to psychotherapy. I look forward to when every healing modality has its own advocates to integrate the science of Memory Reconsolidation.

EMDR and Brainspotting

Psychotherapist David Grand started out using EMDR (Eye Movement Desensitization and Reprocessing) He then discovered a connection between where a person looks, and what memories surface in a person's mind. He's been experimenting and developing ever since. Now over 6,000 therapists have been trained worldwide in the technique of Brainspotting.[59] I read Dr. Grand's book only recently, and with great fascination – from everything he writes the technique he offers is clearly highly effective. And reading with the knowledge of Memory Reconsolidation, I can see that the Brainspotting technique

Integrating ICE with Existing Methods

includes the process of identifying, calming and exchanging. Yet not once in the book did I find any sign that Dr. Grand or any of the trained therapists have yet made the connection to Memory Reconsolidation. The brain science explanation given in the book uses the findings of neuroplasticity and "deep brain" mystery. I found myself excited for the day they incorporate the understanding of Memory Reconsolidation into their experiences.

Coherence Therapy; developed by Ecker, Ticic and Hulley; show us that the Memory Reconsolidation conversation has started. Brainspotting's yet-to-come-awareness of Memory Reconsolidation is an example of how this conversation has only just begun.

The Emotional Freedom Technique (EFT)

EFT also awaits the discovery that their results can be explained by Memory Reconsolidation. The most recent manual of EFT does mention Memory Reconsolidation for the first time, but the three steps of Memory Reconsolidation have not yet been integrated into explaining the EFT method.[60]

I learned EFT some years ago, and the striking effectiveness of this method drove me to start looking for why it works so well. How could people produce such rapid and dramatic changes in their lives? Memory Reconsolidation provided the answer for me. As I noted earlier in this book, I followed the trail and created a technique that mimics as closely as possible the three steps of Memory Reconsolidation. I have a profound debt of gratitude to EFT. I've spoken about Memory Reconsolidation at EFT conferences in Washington and in Canada. Whenever I do, EFT practitioners almost always nod their heads and tell me afterwards, "That makes so much sense. Now I understand what's happening when I use EFT with clients."

Neuromaps

Daimon Sweeney[61] has done more creative work with Memory Reconsolidation than anyone I know. Since he was a youngster he has felt a mission in life. He's committed to helping humanity through what he calls, "this awkward period of our evolution." When he became aware of Memory Reconsolidation his work rose to a whole new level. My favorite innovation of his is something he's named Neuromapping.

Identify an issue you want to work on, then write down everything you can about the issue. Use colors, shapes, connecting lines, whatever you wish. Make a map that represents your current situation. Daimon then has a number of exercises to get your focus off the neuromap and into a place where you produce non-agitated peptides. After one of these exercises, you create a new neuromap to represent how you feel about the issue after doing the exercise. Remarkable changes often occur in a single iteration. Whatever issues remain, or whatever new issues arise, can be addressed by making new neuromaps.

All the other modalities in this chapter show examples of integrating Memory Reconsolidation into already existing practices. Daimon Sweeney's neuromaps show how Memory Reconsolidation can provide the basis for creating an entirely new process. As time goes on I expect more and more methods will arise based directly on the understanding of Memory Reconsolidation.

Quantum Healing

Matrix Energetics[62] and Quantum Entrainment[63] both operate based on our conscious access to the quantum field. These and other quantum methods have similarities to The ICE Method but with the addition of quantum awareness.

A person using a quantum method will typically set an intention or identify an issue in their life. Then without dwelling any longer on that issue they will use an awareness process to create a conscious connection with the quantum field. As I noted in Chapter Ten, I believe that accessing the calm space of nothing corresponds to this awareness of the quantum field. ICE explains itself by referring to material molecules. Quantum explains itself in terms of light, energy and vibration.

After accessing the awareness of the field, the person at some point returns to their "regular" material awareness. Based on the observer effect, this quantum field access often changes the physical and emotional experience of a person's life.

What Memory Reconsolidation might add to quantum methods is the understanding that we can reconsolidate material peptides in the body. If we look back on the exact memories, feelings and body sensations after accessing our awareness of the quantum field, we change our material body and mind. Observing in this way may add to the results that quantum healing already experiences.

It's because we experience a "material" life that Memory Reconsolidation may benefit quantum healing. Peptides show up as long as we live in this human form. Yes, all matter is energy. And yes, peptides can be understood materially or energetically. Memory Reconsolidation can provide a useful bridge between these two worlds of quantum energy and material chemistry.

Native Traditions – Shamanic Methods

> A shaman wants to erase the load of emotions that his or her history carries, to render it neutral. This is what is meant by erasing it. It is helpful to remember that your history is nothing more than a collection of thoughts with emotions attached. When the emotion is gone, the story loses its punch and becomes completely neutral, thus freeing us from feeling compelled to act out (or react) due to these emotions.[64]

So how did people in Native traditions erase the emotions of their memories? "Shamanically speaking, there are various methods of erasing your personal history…what method you use does not matter, as long as it works for you."[65] Ingerman and Wesserman list a number of ways that traditional cultures have used to erase memories. One method involves making lists and recalling items during a breathing exercise. Another method releases memories by rotating one's head or circling or whirling, all the while unwinding the emotions. Certain cultures use hallucinogenic plants while paying attention to memories in a structured way. Others use fire and pay attention to memories in a certain manner.

One of the most dramatic methods is a journey of the spirit called dismemberment. In this spiritual journey the person experiences themselves being taken apart, dismembering and dying in one way or another. Following the dismemberment comes a "re-memberment," or in the terms of this book – a reconsolidation.

Hank Wesserman notes that in workshops he leads,

> A dismemberment journey often marks the end of inflammatory and chronic conditions, even allergies, in which the sufferer emerges healed and

free of formerly debilitating conditions. The frequency of this happening has impressed my inner scientist beyond measure.[66]

If you look closely at any of these methods, they all complete the requirements for Memory Reconsolidation and the replacement of peptides. Any process that completes the steps of identifying an emotional issue, accessing an alternate emotional state and then paying attention to the exact original issue within the four-hour window can cause memories to reconsolidate. Many of our planet's traditional cultures knew about this process. They used it in a wide variety of different methods.

Ingerman and Wesserman compare shamanism to psychotherapy: "Psychoanalysis tries to do the same thing [erasing emotions], but from a shamanic perspective, the psychoanalytic approach tends to reinforce memories because they become such a focus with each session."[67]

Psychoanalyst Bruce Ecker, as mentioned earlier, is well aware of this problem, and his work addresses a solution using the same brain process as traditional cultures used – Memory Reconsolidation.[68]

Today, our respected story is the story of Science. Shamanic traditions sometimes evoke suspicion. So Memory Reconsolidation, coming as a scientific discovery, holds great importance in this conversation. As with quantum science, the recent discoveries of Memory Reconsolidation create the possibility for new bridges between ancient and modern knowings. Memory Reconsolidation already happens in traditional cultures in a variety of practical methods. The scientific discovery of how memories store and restore at the synapse of the brain allows us a deeper way of communicating and learning between cultures.

The Doctor's Office

There's a growing trend towards understanding medicine as "integrative medicine."[69,70] So far that understanding hasn't come to include Memory Reconsolidation, but I look forward to the day it does.

I imagine someday a small Memory Reconsolidation kiosk at the front door of every hospital. Everyone who enters the hospital would receive an ICE Method session or some other modality that helped each patient transform their upsets to calm.

When those kiosks exist, then each patient will visit their doctor from a place of calm cellular chemistry. The cells of each patient's body will be focused on rest, restoration and healing, rather than fight/flight/freeze stress responses. Prescribed medications will be interacting with cells already focused on healing. What a difference from the common experience of medications interacting with bodily stress chemistry.

The kiosks would be used to reconsolidate old stored emotions as well as providing calm in the moment. PTSD and other emotional traumas, panic attacks and anxiety would be resolved at the synaptic level of a patient's brain without resorting to anxiety medications or other prescribed chemical interventions.

Memory Reconsolidation kiosks. Keep your eye out for when the first one arrives at your local hospital. Until then, find someone who understands the transformative emotional and physical benefits that Memory Reconsolidation can provide. If you find something better than The ICE Method, I'll be happy for you. If you don't, the process here in this book allows you to get started right now.

14 – Last Words

I still remember my excitement when I first became aware of Memory Reconsolidation. "Really?" I thought to myself, "This is the way our minds work?"

Tons of complexity and mystery surround neuroscience, but the concept of Memory Reconsolidation can be simply grasped, understood, and employed.

**Identify. Calm. Exchange peptides.
Transform lives.**

I've been privileged to stand alongside such a variety of people and watch them start using The ICE Method in their lives. I've watched physical issues, emotional issues and spiritual issues transform to calm, peace and health. While this doesn't happen every single time, it does far more than I would ever have believed possible.

Ten years from now. Maybe five. Memory Reconsolidation will someday have its place in regular public conversation. Radio DJ's will share human interest shorts of people who found calm in their lives, when all they'd had before was trauma. Doctors will explore how chronic diseases can dissipate when stored emotional peptides become calm. Individuals and families will discover the impact Memory Reconsolidation can have on their history and on their daily experience of life. I look forward to when the world spins this way.

In these last few words of this book, let me try to clearly distinguish between the *me* in The ICE Method and the *mechanical process* of The ICE Method.

- Much of what I love about The ICE Method is that people can learn the technique and do the mechanics of ICE immediately. Identify. Calm. Exchange. Do this, and you're doing Memory Reconsolidation.

- As you gain familiarity with ICE, you learn of deeper ways to identify stored upset peptides. Again, anyone can do this.
- When people tell me "You're so skilled at this," I respond first by explaining the above two points. And then I explain my skill is like Goldilocks who finds a chair that hopefully fits "just right" and a bowl of porridge that tastes "just right."

If peptides get activated too intensely a person can go into dissociation (Chapter Eight). I help people keep those peptides activating at a rate that feels "just right." This is a skill, a sensitivity, a way of listening and a way of being. I have this skill. Without it you can still do The ICE Method. With it you will get better results with less dissociation. The experience will feel smoother for people.

If peptides don't activate they can't reconsolidate. I help people make connections from one part of their life to another, thus activating peptides sooner than they otherwise might. I help people keep those peptides activating at a rate that works "just right" for them. This too is a skill. Without it you can still do The ICE Method. With it you will get faster and more comprehensive results.

So when I facilitate people to experience The ICE Method, both parts work; the mechanical process, and my personal presence in the process. I enjoy being a part of this with people. Yes, I'm pleased to acknowledge that I consider myself good at this work. And I insist on pointing out you don't have to be me to do ICE – ICE offers a mechanical process you can start using immediately – and when you do, your skills will start increasing.

I currently work as a part of The Integrative Medical Clinic at Wellness Gardens here in Chelan, Washington. I share The ICE Method with a wide variety of people. When the time arrives that Memory Reconsolidation becomes widely known, I hope ICE will continue to serve as a useful tool. If ICE remains relevant and does have a role to play, I'll look forward to finding broader ways to share The ICE Method and train others who want to use it. Or perhaps when Memory Reconsolidation really gets rolling another method will develop that provides even quicker and more effective results. If that happens, I'll go get whatever training becomes available. What I want most is to continue helping others receive the gift of calm and peace that Memory Reconsolidation can so effectively provide.

A wonderful journey lies ahead, seeing how Memory Reconsolidation unfolds into our public awareness. Now you have your eyes open too, so we can watch and participate together.

Before it came to be, I never ever thought that sharing The ICE Method would be my life. Now I help people experience their own transformation of mind, body and spirit. I feel beyond thankful. If The ICE Method matches what you truly want for your life, then I hope that Memory Reconsolidation will also come to live with you at the center of your being, at the center of your journey.

Transforming wishes for identifying, calming and exchanging the peptides of your life.

Workbook and Journal

This book you just read can get you off to a great start using The ICE Method.

The Workbook and Journal can provide you additional benefits.

Working with a wide variety of people helped me experiment and find effective ways for people to reconsolidate emotional upsets. The workbook shares a series of exercises you can follow as a guide for reconsolidating your own memories. The exercises start out with reconsolidating one of your specific memories. The workbook then gradually guides you to ICE'ing your Download and other foundational memories. The final extended section provides an exercise for reconsolidating high-intensity upsets such as PTSD and abuse.

Gain ICE Method proficiency quicker.

If you use the workbook, you'll get all my experience at your fingertips. With the workbook you can start out living The ICE Method life at a much higher level. From this level, you can more easily work on your own life, and the lives of other people. If you choose to work with others, you'll find yourself developing your own style, and maybe even a completely distinct technique. Whatever direction you take with The ICE Method, this workbook will greatly accelerate your journey.

As I say to the people I work with when they ask what's next: "Everything is next. Go ICE everything that feels upset." Those who take this to heart gain a transformed life.

Order your workbook at *MemoryReconsolidationApplied.com* or directly from Amazon.

Personal Sessions and Coaching

When I'm not tucked away writing about The ICE Method, I work collaboratively at Wellness Gardens Integrative Medical Center here in Chelan, Washington. I facilitate the ICE Method for individuals and for groups. I provide in-person sessions for those who live in Central Washington. I offer online or phone sessions for those living farther away.

For a limited number of clients, I offer personal ICE Method coaching. Some people use me as a coach for working through difficult issues in their life. Some people see me for chronic pain issues. Others have started the journey to a life of calm, and they want a guide to help them stop living their old life of constant reactivity and emotional upset.

If you're drawn in the direction of helping others, contact me and I'll be glad to assist you, either through personal sessions or as your personal coach. Check the website for ICE Method training workshops and programs.

Author

"He's a case. He's more than most people have to deal with." Seattle Evening Magazine had arrived to film my unicycle ride from Mexico to Canada. The camera captured this moment as my wife Anne shared her description of me. We have laughed about this story a hundred times – the description still seems to fit.

Anne and I first met in 1983, just after I completed a mechanical engineering degree at Cal Berkeley. She missed out on my time at the Air Force Academy in Colorado. By the time we got married I was in seminary studying to be a Lutheran pastor. We did my internship in Alaska after a six-month honeymoon on a tandem bike in Europe. I served my first church in Nome, Alaska – a life changing experience of living in a hunting-gathering culture at the interface with Western culture. Our son and daughter were born here.

The next church was right in the middle of American culture – campus ministry at Michigan State University. The student population of 40,000 numbered ten times the city of Nome. In the year 2000 I left ordained ministry, and we moved to Whidbey Island in the Puget Sound of Washington – which led to a unicycle ride through all fifty states – which led to living in the heart of the Cascade Mountains for two years, in a community accessible only by boat up Lake Chelan – which led to ten years of living here in Chelan – our longest time in one place together, by far.

My first two books shared unicycling adventures. *One Wheel – Many Spokes* tells about the fifty-state ride that set two Guinness World Records. After that I rode 1500 miles through the Northeast states, asking people their opinions about a subject that was more contentious back in 2004 – rights for gay and lesbian, bisexual, and transgender people. I published *Straight Into Gay America* after that ride.

I never expected to spend my days helping people heal from emotional and physical distress, but I'm glad for this life. It's a rare day

I don't walk through this town of 4,000 people without running into someone I've helped to learn and use The ICE Method.

During these last ten years Anne and I have also developed a fascination for growing food and living with an eye toward sustainability. I manage a community garden with 40 wonderful volunteers, one of the most delightful places to spend time. I think we may have finally settled down…

Appendix – The Field

Quantum provides an optional but valuable addition for understanding our experiences. If you already know about quantum, I expect you feel as excited as me about how Memory Reconsolidation fits with quantum. If you find yourself engaging quantum for the first time, you may find your world flipping upside down – as it has for me and so many who have engaged quantum science.

In this appendix we'll look at three experiments that give us a whole new view of how the world works. The two conclusions from these experiments are:

> **Everything is Connected.**
> **and "What We *Get* is What We *See*."**

Everything is Connected

Have you ever had a friend visit, and when they leave to drive away, you realize you forgot to tell them something? So you start running after their car, but they drive too fast: you can't catch up. That's what happens in the Classical or Newtonian world, the world of our everyday experience. In the quantum world, you can catch up.

Non-Locality

Just like the two friends visiting, imagine two subatomic particles, joined as a pair. When these particles come together, it's like they can have a close "conversation." In physics terms this conversation is called "spin." When one particle spins in one direction, the other particle always adapts to spin in the other direction. You can view spin like smiley faces. In terms of subatomic particles, if one smiles the other frowns. When one switches, the other one also switches right away.

Now, just like your friend who drove away, scientists took two paired smiley face particles and separated them. One of the particles they kept at "home." The other one they let "drive" away at the speed of light. Remember in the example of the car – you couldn't catch up. What about the particles, though? Remember that these particles were paired. When they were together, if you changed one from a smile to a frown, the other one had to change in response, immediately.

Researchers wanted to know what would happen to the drive-away smiley face when you changed the one that had stayed at home. So, they changed the particle at home from a smile to a frown. What happened to the smiley face that had traveled far away?

That other smiley face particle was traveling at the speed of light. In our normal classical (or Newtonian) understanding, this is the fastest anything can travel, 176,000 miles per second. So, of course the spin change from the smiley at home couldn't ever catch up to the far away frown. And yet, when the home particle changed from a smile to a frown, the far-away particle reacted instantly. The information did catch up and the far away smiley face *immediately* changed from a frown to a smile.

This experiment showed an incredible fact, that information really can travel faster than the speed of light. In fact it takes no time at all to travel. Information can transmit instantly, regardless of distance.

Scientists call this "non-locality."

**Information can transmit instantaneously
without the limitations of time or space.**

This experiment was first carried out in 1997, and has been repeated many times since. I remember first reading about it when I was serving as a campus pastor at Michigan State University. Right away I started thinking about prayer differently than I ever had before. In fact, I started thinking about everything differently. Ever since first reading about non-locality, I have thought about the world in a much more connected way. Physicist Menas Kafatos calls the discovery of non-locality, "the most momentous in the history of science."[71] For a great description of this experiment and the ones in the next section, see Chapter Eight of Robert Lanza's *Biocentrism.*[72]

Entanglement

Non-locality experiments are predicted by theory. Experiments have measured the effect with two paired subatomic particles. Would the experiment work with three particles? With four? Of course. And you and I, at least in a material sense, are just a larger collection of subatomic particles.

Some scientists hesitate to say that humans function as quantum beings. Even Einstein hesitated. The experiments show a world so different from traditional material science that one can understand the reluctance. These quantum findings seem closer to spiritual experience than the science of Newton and Descartes. Given the contest between science and religion these past 300 years, no wonder some scientists have held back. And yet, holding back from quantum doesn't make sense. If two subatomic particles act non-locally then, of course, trillions of particles would also act this way. Scientists who do see these connections call this the "entangled" universe. And we humans are entangled right in with it.

In the entangled universe, everything is connected across all time and across all space.

In fact, even time and space are not needed to make the mathematical equations of quantum mechanics work. Time and space are constructs we use to make sense of our material universe.

A related word for entanglement is the "holographic" universe. In a hologram the entire universe is contained in every smaller piece of the universe. Mind boggling – yes – but go back to the two smiley faces that instantly know and react when a change is made to the other face, even at a distance. Keep adding smiley faces to the experiment until you have every particle in the universe. Now everything is entangled so every part of the universe has instantaneous communication with every other part of the universe. This is a hologram. Implications for healing, anyone?

Okay, so we live in a non-local universe, an entangled universe, a hologram. That provides plenty to absorb. It also turns out that things in the universe show up depending on how we look at them, specifically *whether or not* we are looking at them, observing them.

What we *get* is what we *see*.

Particle or Wave?

In an early quantum experiment over a hundred years ago, scientists wondered whether light was a wave or whether light was a particle. They set up this experiment called "the double-slit" experiment and started firing photons (the smallest units of light) through the experiment. As they watched, the photons showed themselves to be particles, behaving like baseballs a boy might pitch at a target for practice.

Later, for whatever reason, the scientists ran the experiment again, but this time they didn't watch. Maybe they needed a coffee break and forgot to turn off the photon beam. When they came back to check on their little baseballs - amazement. It appeared as if the boy had stopped throwing balls at the target. The scientists found that when they didn't watch the experiment, the photons behaved like waves instead of particles.[73]

Scientists have repeated this experiment hundreds of times, and the result always remains the same. Watch the experiment and light behaves like a baseball pitcher throwing strikes. Don't watch the experiment and light behaves like a wave, like a ripple on a pond. It turns out the only thing that matters is whether or not you observe the experiment while the beam throws photons. Observe the photons and you get material particles; baseballs. Don't observe the photons and you get a wave pattern; a "probability" of possibilities.

Once again, if this experiment works for single photons of light, it should also work for many subatomic particles together. If you take all the photons and subatomic particles together you get a really strange universe.

**Only while you look
does the thing appear there as a solid object.**

When you don't look, it's a wave form that contains all probabilities.

Only when you're looking

While you look, during the time you observe, scientists call this "collapsing the wave." You collapse the situation from all possibilities down to the single one you observe. A tree is a tree when you look at it

– *only* when you look at it. When you're not looking, it's the potential of tree or many other things.

No matter how long scientists have been involved with quantum, they end up using the word "weird," when they describe its effects. As a child, and even as a college student, no one told me the world works in this quantum way.

As an example; grab a carton of milk from the refrigerator and pour some on your cereal. When you put it back in the refrigerator and stop looking at it, the milk now exists as a wave of probabilities. And yet you can tell your partner where the milk is and he can open the cooler and get the milk, too. And the milk came from someone observing cow and putting that cow in the milking barn a few days earlier. No wonder the scientists call this weird – and yet, according to the math, and according to the experiments; on the quantum level the world works this way. Entanglement. Hologram. Observer Effect.

Non-local Observation

Okay, so here's where we're going.

We're going to take the non-local smiley face finding from the last chapter and combine it with the baseball/wave observer effect from this chapter. This will give us something very useful to The ICE Method.

Then we'll look at how these quantum findings can combine with Memory Reconsolidation and peptides. We'll see how this can make a difference for healing.

Let's see what happens when you combine entanglement with the observer effect – combining smiley faces and baseballs.

The experiment

First, set up two of the double slit baseball/wave experiments. Now shoot the paired smiley faces through each of these double slit experiments. Send all the smiles through one of the experiments, and send all the paired frown faces through the other experiment. In this way you combine the baseball experiment (waves vs. particles) with the smiley face experiment (spin information can travel infinitely fast.) In this experiment frowns and smiles travel the same distance and strike their receptors at the same time. Send a whole stream of smile faces and frown faces through the experiment and see what you get.

Observation

If you *observe* one side of the experiment, let's say the smiling faces, you will see that these faces will act like particles, like baseballs thrown at a target. If you fire the smiling faces through the experiment *without observing* it, you get wave behavior.

Observing one experiment affects the other

Interestingly, whatever you do to one side of the experiment, the other side will do the same thing – because these smiley faces are entangled.

- If the smiley face appears like a particle on the one side, the frown face hitting the other receiver will also appear as a particle. Remember – when you watch something it appears as a particle, and when you watch one particle it affects the other particle.
- Also remember – when you don't observe the experiment you get wave behavior. So, if you don't observe the smiley faces on the one experiment, they will form a wave pattern and so will the frown faces going through the other experiment.

So, again:

**because the particles are paired,
whatever you do to the one affects the other.**

In this experiment you get the instantaneous communication between two paired particles, and you also get the particle/wave behavior that results from observing or not observing the experiment. Take your time absorbing this – for most of us its new ground – I kept turning this over in my head for a long time before it started making some sense to me.

Backwards in time

Okay, if you feel ready, let's do one last modification. This experiment was first done in 2002.[74] This result showed that effects can take place *backwards* in time.

Take the same two double slit detectors for this experiment. Next take one of them and move it much farther from the particle source. Now when you run the experiment, the smiley particle gets to the close detector before the frown particle gets to the distant detector.

Appendix - The Field

If no one watches this experiment, both receptor plates again exhibit wave behavior. From the previous experiments we would expect this to happen.

If an observer watches the closer receptor then they will see particles at that receptor. And since the particles are paired, the distant receptor also appears like particles.

What happens when you observe the distant receptor but *not* the closer receptor?

The distant receptor, if you watch it, shows up like particles, like baseballs. Let's say that all the smiley faces got sent to this distant receptor. The question for the experimenters was, "What happens to the frown faces at the close receptor."

Again, take your time with this. At the closer receptor the frown faces have *already* completed their journey before the smiley faces landed. And no one had watched the frown faces, so they should be like waves, right? Remember, if you don't watch, you get wave behavior. If you do watch you get particle behavior. The distant smiley faces were observed only *after* the nearby frowns already landed. So, what happened?

In this experiment, the unobserved photons did not form a wave – they behaved as particles, like baseballs.

When the distant particles were observed, this had an effect on the smiley faces that had *already* landed. Even though no one had watched these baseballs land, they turned up as particles. When the smiles changed to frowns in the distant receptor, the frown faces that had already landed still changed to smiles – even though no one watched them land! This result happened *backwards in time!*

In this experiment, the observer effect and entanglement created a result *backwards* in time!

Memory Reconsolidation Applied

Here's a direct application to Memory Reconsolidation. With The ICE Method we constantly go back in time to replace stored emotional upsets with calm peptides. If you think in terms of this experiment, we make a new observation at a later time, sometimes even decades later. And this observation changes what we first observed back at the time of the experience, the original upset. In one sense, ICE is like changing the spin of those frown faces to the smiley faces. The ICE Method can be visualized either as material peptides, or else in this alternative way. The ICE Method can be understood in terms of the quantum observer effect and quantum entanglement.

Okay, if you haven't had any exposure to quantum before, I hope you find yourself fascinated. You can discover all sorts of great resources to learn and explore more about the field. Hopefully this introduction will help you make better sense of Chapter Ten and how quantum and ICE can go together.

Remember, you don't need to understand any of this to experience the relief of symptoms that comes from identifying, calming and exchanging peptides so your old upset emotions can reconsolidate to calm. That remains the single main point of this whole book. Quantum can add a lot to our understanding, but you can do ICE without any quantum knowledge. If you find quantum frustrating, you can ICE it all to calm, and then get back to your calm life! Good wishes.

Disclaimer

Lars Clausen is not a medical doctor. He holds a Master's Degree in Mechanical Engineering and earned a Master of Divinity Degree preceding his service as a pastor. Lars Clausen does not offer medical advice. He uses the non-invasive ICE Method to work with people who bring emotional or physical issues for relief. Lars Clausen is not responsible for clients' experience with The ICE Method or their results.

The ICE Method is not traditional Western medicine – it is not medicine. The hypothesis is that the ICE Method works by invoking an awareness of emotional responses engaging neuropeptides in the process of memory reconsolidation. In this process the body and mind will often experience relief. The ICE Method is in an experimental stage. You must use your own common sense in deciding the appropriateness of The ICE Method for you. If you have any medical or other questions about using The ICE Method, you should consult with your health care provider before using it or scheduling a session.

The ICE Method does not guarantee either specific or general outcomes for clients. The contents of this book make no guarantee as to accuracy or results. All content is the personal opinion of Lars Clausen and is not medical or psychological advice. Usage of any content is the responsibility of the reader.

Index

A

Abby - Chronic Fatigue Syndrome 93
Acupunture 157
Alcoholics Anonymous 124
Allergies 137
Appendix 175
Author 173
Autoimmunity 136

B

Ben's Story - Anger 19
Birthright Calm 101, 143
Body 52
Brain wiring 121
Brainspotting 160
Bruce Ecker 124

C

Calm xi, xii, 20, 23, 24, 34, 46, 51, 53, 55, 74, 75, 85, 87, 95, 97, 101, 111, 123, 125, 129, 131, 136, 139, 140, 143
Calm beach 64
Candace Pert .... xii, 22, 35
Catherine Freeman 157
Christian Worship 157
Coaching 172
Coherence Therapy 124, 159
Compassion 143
Confession and Forgiveness 158
Consciousness 138
Counteractive therapy 124
Craniosacral Therapy 155
Culture 98

D

Daimon Sweeney 161
Danish soldiers 114
David Grand 160
Death 151
Disclaimer xv
Dissociation 61, 106, 110
Doctor 164
Dorthe Berntson 113
Download 76, 87

E

Ecker, Bruce 124
EFT .... xii, 31, 33, 41, 161
Einstein 134
EMDR 160
Emotion 51
Emotional Freedom Technique ..... xii, 31, 33, 41, 161
Emotional pain 81
Emotions 47
Energy Ball 131
Entanglement 176
Exchange 54

F

Fibromyalgia 38, 47
Fibromyalgia Study 72
Fight/flight/freeze . xii, 22, 23, 39, 47, 51, 53, 54, 61, 74, 78, 114, 136
Focus 95
Frank Kinslow 48
Freedom 145

Freeman, Catherine 157
Fritz Albert Popp 135

G

Ginevra Liptan 47
Goldilocks 168
Grand, David 160

H

Habit 121
Hospital 164

I

ICE Method . xi, xii, xv, 19, 34, 48, 51, 71, 74, 75, 85, 101, 110, 113, 131, 138, 139, 144, 148, 167
    Quantum 128
ICE'ing the ancestors 101
ICE'ing Womb Time 100
Identify 51
Integrative Medical Clinic 168
Intention 133
Inupiat Eskimo 98

J

James - Spiders 31
James Pennebaker 156
Jeff - Frozen Shoulder 41
Jeff - Panic Attack 115
John Neff 156
Joseph LeDoux 33, 34
Journal 171
Journaling 155

K

Karim Nader .... xiii, 40
Kim Levinson -The Light Within 130
Kinslow, Frank 48
Kyrie 158

L

Lars - hamstring 81

LeDoux, Joseph 33, 34
Levinson, Kim 130
Light Within 130
Liptan, Ginevra 47
Long-distance healing 133
Lynn - Chronic Pain 75, 89

M

Manifesting 84, 85
Massage 154
Meditational practice 139
Memory Reconsolidation. xiii, 20, 33, 34, 37, 45
Molecules of Emotion 35
Mountain visualization 111
Movie test 32, 101
Multiple Sclerosis 136

N

Nader, Karim .... xiii, 40
Neff, John 156
Neurogenesis 121
Neuromaps 161
Neuroplasticity 121
Nome, Alaska 98
Non-attachment .... xiv, 75, 140, 144
Non-local 179
Non-Locality 135, 175
Nothing 47
Number anxiety 115

O

Observer effect 127, 178

P

Palumbo, Paul 158
Particle 178
Paul Palumbo 158
Pennebaker, James 156
Penny - PTSD 61
Personal Sessions 172
Pert, Candace 22, 35
Popp, Fritz Albert 135
Psychotheraphy 159

182

PTSD 105, 110, 111

Q

Qi Gong 156

R

Reactivity 78
Religion 138

S

Sandra Ingerman 147
Sarah - Fibromyalgia 38
Secondary Gain 77
Shaman 147
Spiritual practice 139
Stress 22, 25, 38, 53, 74, 86, 95, 96, 115, 136, 158
Structural pain 81
Subsequent Rounds 55
Sweeney, Daimon 161
Synapse 35, 63

T

The Field 175
The ICE Method xi, xii, xv, 19, 34, 48, 51, 71, 74, 75, 85, 101, 110, 113, 131, 138, 139, 144, 148, 167
Theta brain wave 86, 98
Theta wave state 144, 146
Three-step dance 55
Tigers 80, 96
Time 180

U

Unlocking the Emotional Brain 159

V

Vibrations 135

W

Wave 178
What you *want* 71, 74
Workarounds 122
Workbook 171

Z

Zero Point Field 134

Endnotes

[1] C. Alberini, Memory Reconsolidation, (London, Academic Press, 2013).
[2] B. Ecker, R Ticic, L. Hulley, Unlocking the Emotional Brain, (New York, Routledge, 2012).
[3] L. Clausen, Fibromyalgia Relief: A Science-Based Approach to Healing Body, Mind, and Spirit. (CreateSpace 2013).
[4] C. Pert, Molecules of Emotion, (New York, Scribner, 1997).
[5] J. LeDoux, The Synaptic Self: How Our Brains Become Who We Are, (New York, Penguin, 2002) 161.
[6] Alberini.
[7] Pert.
[8] B. Lipton, The Biology of Belief, (Carlsbad, California, Hay House, 2008) Ch. 6.
[9] F. Kinslow, The Secret of Instant Healing (USA, Lucid Sea, 2008).
[10] D. Schiller, M. Monfils, et al. "Preventing the return of fear in humans using reconsolidation update mechanisms," Nature Vol 463, Issue 7277 (2010): doi:10.1038/nature 08637.
[11] B. Ecker, R Ticic, L. Hulley, Unlocking the Emotional Brain, (New York, Routledge, 2012)
[12] D. Sweeney, www.NeuromasteryAcademy.com.
[13] Clausen, 83-85.
[14] G. Craig, The EFT Manual, (Energy Psychology Press, 2011).
[15] LeDoux, 161.
[16] Pert.
[17] S. Chen, C. Shanping; et al. "Reinstatement of long-term memory following erasure of its behavioral and synaptic expression in Aplysia" eLife Journal, (November, 2014) elifesciences.org/content/3/e03896.
[18] Pert.
[19] Pert, 145.
[20] Pert, 189.
[21] Alberini – Kindle Location 348.

[22] K. Nader, G. Schafe, J. LeDoux, "Fear memories require protein synthesis in the amygdala for reconsolidation after retrieval." Nature, (2000): (ncbi.nlm.nih.gov/pubmed/10963596)

[23] Schiller.

[24] R. Callahan, Tapping the Healer Within: Using Thought-Field Therapy to Instantly Conquer Your Fears, Anxieties, and Emotional Distress, (New York, McGraw-Hill, 2002).

[25] G. Liptan, Figuring Out Fibromyalgia (Portland OR, Visceral Press, 2011).

[26] Liptan, 28.

[27] Liptan, 56.

[28] Liptan, 20.

[29] Kinslow.

[30] Lipton, Ch. 6.

[31] D. Church, G. Yount, A Brooks, "Psychological Trauma Symptom Improvements in Veterans Using Emotional Freedom Technique: A Randomized Controlled Trial" Journal of Nervous and Mental Diseases 201(2) (2013): 153-160.

[32] National Institute of Mental Health (nimh.nih.gov/health/topics/post-traumatic-stress-disorder-ptsd/index.shtml).

[33] D.C. Rubin, D. Berntsen, M.K. Johansen, "A Memory Based Model of Postraumatic Stress Disorder: Evaluating Basic Assumptions Underlying the PTSD Diagnosis Psychological Review 115(4) (2008) 985-1011.

[34] D. Berntsen, K.B. Johannesen, Y.D. Thomsen, M. Bertelsen, R.H. Hoyles, D.C. Rubin, "Peace and War: Trajectories of Posttraumatic Stress Disorder Symptoms Before, During, and After Military Deployment in Afghanistan," Psychological Science, (2012) pss.sagepub.com/content/23/12/1557.

[35] W. Herbert, "Troubled Childhood May Predict PTSD," Scientific American Mind, 23(5) (2012).

[36] Aarhus University, "War is not necessarily the cause of post-traumatic disorder," Science Daily, August 17, 2012) sciencedaily.com/releases/2012/08/120817135532.htm.

[37] Clausen.

[38] J. Dispenza, Evolve Your Brain: The Science of Changing Your Mind, (Health Communications, 2007).

[39] Ecker, 14.

[40] M. Dahlitz, "Editors Notes." The Psychoneurotherapist, 11 (2015)

[41] L. McTaggart, The Field, (New York, Harper, 2008) 19.

[42] McTaggart, 39-53.

43 G. Mate, When the Body Says No, (Wiley, 2011).
44 R. Lanza.
45 T. Campell, My Big Toe, (Lightning Strike Books, 2007).
46 S. Ingerman, H. Wesserman, Awakening to the Spirit World: The Shamanic Path of Direct Revelation, (ISA. Sounds True, 2010) 30.
47 Ingerman, 16.
48 Campbell.
49 Ingerman, 11.
50 Ingerman, 11.
51 Ingerman, 13.
52 Ingerman, 13.
53 J. Pennebaker, Writing to Heal, (New Harbinger Publications 2004).
54 J. Neff, www.deepspringwellness.com.
55 C. Freeman, www.acupuncturegarden.com.
56 P. Palumbo, In Defense of the Pastor, (CreateSpace 2013).
57 Ecker.
58 Ecker, 3.
59 D. Grand, Brainspotting: The Revolutionary New Therapy for Rapid and Effective Change, (Boulder, True Sounds 2013).
60 D. Church The EFT Manual (Energy Psychology Press. Kindle Edition. 2013) Kindle Location 773.
61 Sweeney.
62 R. Bartlett, Matrix Energetics (Atria Books/Beyond Words, 2007).
63 Kinslow.
64 Ingerman, 220.
65 Ingerman, 221.
66 Ingerman, 217.
67 Ingerman, 222.
68 Ecker, 3, 14.
69 L. Wisneski, The Scientific Basis of Integrative Medicine, (USA, CRC Press 2009).
70 R. Anderson, Stories of Healing: A Family Doctor's Journal, (Everett WA., Starseed 2011).
71 Nadeau.
72 R. Lanza, Biocentrism, (BenBella Books, 2010) Chapter 8.
73 Lanza, Chapter 8.
74 Lanza, Chapter 8.

Printed in Great Britain
by Amazon